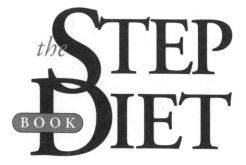

the STEP DIET BOOK

COUNT STEPS, NOT CALORIES, *to* LOSE WEIGHT *and* KEEP IT OFF FOREVER

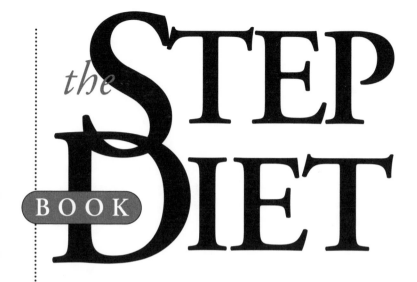

the STEP DIET

BOOK

James O. Hill, Ph.D.,
John C. Peters, Ph.D.,
with Bonnie T. Jortberg, M.S., R.D.

Foreword by Pamela M. Peeke, M.D., M.P.H.

Workman Publishing · New York

Library of Congress Cataloging-in-Publication data

The step diet book: count steps, not calories, to lose weight and keep it off forever.
James O. Hill, John C. Peters, Bonnie T. Jortberg.
p. cm.
ISBN 0-7611-3324-0 (alk. paper)
1. Weight loss. 2. Walking. 3. Reducing diets. I. Hill, James O. II. Peters, John C.
III. Jortberg, Bonnie T.

RM222.2.S7775 2004
613.7'12—dc22   2004046452

Workman books are available at special discounts when purchased in bulk for premiums and sales promotions as well as for fund-raising or educational use. Special editions or book excerpts can also be created to specification. For details, contact the Special Sales Director at the address below.

Workman Publishing Company, Inc.
708 Broadway
New York, NY 10003-9555
www.workman.com

Printed in U.S.A.
10 9 8 7 6 5 4 3 2 1

Acknowledgments

Does the world really need another diet book? We asked ourselves that question dozens of times before deciding to write *The Step Diet Book.* We answered yes when we realized that, despite the hundreds of books available on dieting, most people remain confused about what it takes to gain control of their own weight. This book is our attempt to communicate the truths we have learned about weight management over the past twenty-five years—truths we don't think you are hearing in other books.

We wish we could guarantee that every one of you who reads *The Step Diet Book* will achieve and maintain his or her dream weight, but you wouldn't believe us if we did. So, instead of offering a guarantee, allow us to offer hope: People who use the information and strategies provided here *can* control their weight. Indeed, many of you *will* succeed, possibly beyond your wildest dreams. We wish you good luck.

We have learned from many people. The participants in the National Weight Control Registry have taught us so much about what it takes to keep weight off permanently. These wonderful individuals have learned how to take control of their own energy balance and their own weight, and should be great inspiration for everyone who reads this book. We owe a great debt to the National Institutes of Health for funding twenty-five years of our weight management research. The staff of the Center for Human Nutrition at the University of Colorado has been extremely supportive of our work, and the Procter & Gamble Company has graciously allowed Dr. Peters to work on this project. Finally, we sincerely thank our families for providing encouragement, support, and understanding throughout this project.

This book is dedicated
to those who have lost weight and
kept it off permanently—
and to all the many more
who have the power within them
to join those esteemed ranks.

Contents

FOREWORD

Most mornings when I wake up, there's a brief moment when I engage in a mind-over-mattress dialogue. Should I get up and take that walk, or fall back into that feathered pillow and succumb to the tempting comfort and warmth of my blankets? The bed looks pretty good. But, then, so do my slim-fitting Calvin Klein jeans. If I don't walk, I'll not only start packing on the pounds, pop out of my pants, and look and feel miserable, but I'll eventually get diseases I could have prevented. Nope. Game over. I'm doing the walking thing. Sleepy-eyed, I eventually achieve the vertical, hop into my sweats and sneakers, strap my pedometer to my waistband, and head out to walk. Like putting money in a piggy bank, I start to accrue my daily steps. Why? Because Jim Hill and John Peters told me to.

So, just who are these guys and why do they have such power and control over my life?

Well, for one thing, they're the wizards of walking, the A Team of the science of weight control and fitness—two of the most powerful voices in obesity research in the country. And now, thank heavens, they've finally written a book to explain how anyone can literally take that first step to a longer, happier, and healthier life—and a slimmer one at that!

I've had the distinct pleasure of knowing the dynamic duo of Hill and Peters for over a decade. We share a passion for translating cutting-edge science (and they've done a lot of it) into easy-to-digest information for people who want to achieve and maintain an optimal body for life. *The Step Diet Book,* which is all about taking the simplest steps to stop weight gain, does this and more. Who can't move 100 calories more each day and eat 100 calories less? And once you've seen that you can stop that speeding train of weight gain, how about losing the weight? Not a problem. Hill and Peters have teamed up with the highly talented nutritionist Bonnie Jortberg to create an innovative roadmap to weight loss that teaches us to balance what we eat with getting up and moving more. With this book, they have put the concept of "energy balance" on the map.

As you'll see when you read *The Step Diet Book,* getting the weight off and keeping it off are two distinct processes. How do we know this? Because of Jim Hill's brilliant work at the University of Colorado, supervising the country's only large-scale study of "successful losers" in the National Weight Control Registry. More than 3,000 participants who have shed at least 30 pounds and kept it off for many years have taught Hill and his co-workers what it takes to make weight control a lifetime success story for each of us. That too is all about small, realistic changes that anyone can do, and this book will tell you how.

In case you don't know it (and I bet you do), we're in the midst of the greatest health care threat to ever hit this country—the obesity epidemic. Here are some wake-up-and-hear-the-warning stats:

- The recent Surgeon General's report said 27 percent of Americans are obese, and 61 percent are overweight.

- Obesity exacts a higher toll on health and health care costs than either smoking or drinking.

- A recent study found that obesity, which is linked to health complications including diabetes, arthritis, heart disease, stroke, and certain cancers, raises a person's health care costs by 36 percent and medication costs by 77 percent.

- Being obese at age twenty can cut up to twenty years off a person's life.

- The National Cancer Institute notes that 14 percent of cancer deaths in men and 20 percent of cancer deaths in women might be due to being overweight or obese.

- Among more than 9,500 Americans surveyed, obesity was associated with higher rates of chronic medical problems and a poorer quality of life than were alcohol abuse, smoking, and poverty.

- In 1990, 11.4 percent of Americans were obese. By the year 2000, that number had risen to 19.6 percent. It is estimated that close to 40 percent of Americans will be obese by the year 2010.

- Researchers have discovered that obese children already show unhealthy changes in their arteries, which increase the risk of health problems later in life.

Drs. Hill and Peters have heard this call to arms and in response have written a remarkable book. (This is also why they've created a national nonprofit initiative called America on the Move™ that you may have heard about.) As all of you are painfully aware, there's so much confusing information out there. Cut the calories, eat whatever you want, eat only fruit, run from carbs, mix and match your foods, exercise fast, move it slower—no wonder we're not getting anywhere. The solution? Simple. Listen to the real scientists who have done the hottest, most current research tell you how to do it. Jim Hill and John Peters have given you the gift of an easy-to-read, realistic, and doable program. Now lace up those walking shoes and start moving today. It may be the biggest step you've ever taken.

PAMELA M. PEEKE, M.D., M.P.H.
Pew Foundation Scholar in Nutrition and Metabolism,
Assistant Professor of Medicine, University of Maryland School of Medicine,
Author of Fight Fat After Forty

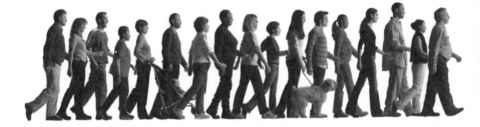

Introduction

Unless you live on a desert island, you are well aware that many of us are too heavy, and that this trend shows no signs of reversing itself. How can this be, you may wonder, with all the "miracle diets" to choose from? Lose 20 pounds in twenty days! Watch fat melt away like magic! You've seen the ads, you've listened to "diet doctors" reveal their secrets on talk shows, perhaps you've tried a fad diet or two. Some of these diets can give you dramatic results, but most focus on quick weight loss rather than long-term weight control. They are not based on sound scientific research. What good is losing 20 pounds in three weeks if you gain it back two months later? Obviously, your real goal should be to maintain whatever weight loss you achieve—and to achieve that loss with a plan that's good for your overall health.

Most diets ultimately fail because they provide a temporary solution, not a permanent way to live your life at a lower weight. But there *is* a way to lose weight without giving those excess pounds a round-trip ticket. The Step Diet is based on scientific research conducted by us and by other researchers. We have studied not just how to lose weight, but how to make small, permanent changes in your lifestyle to keep that weight off forever. And it's easy to get started—all you have to do is put one foot in front of the other.

Count Your Steps

Are you ready to make your first move toward permanent weight loss? Then take out the step counter that came with this book and clip it on your waist (to your belt, pants, or underwear). You have just begun the Step Diet, a scientifically based, people-tested, easy-to-follow program that will take you step by step toward successful weight management. Much more than a plan for simply losing weight, the Step Diet is about overcoming the environmental influences that trigger weight gain so you can keep the weight off. It is about putting you in control of sustaining a body weight that is healthy and right for you. It is about starting where you are right now and making small lifestyle changes that will put you in control of your own weight.

We know from experience that most people can learn to control their weight. Many of us are capable of losing some weight and keeping it off for good. Others can still learn to avoid gaining the 1 to 2 pounds that most adults put on each year. Whatever your specific goal, keep in mind that you did not lose control of your weight overnight, and you won't get it back overnight. But with the Step Diet, you can start managing your weight more effectively right now—and from now on.

A Different Approach to Weight Management

It's actually not all that hard to lose weight; you just reduce the amount of food you eat. Why, then, do so many people fail at long-term weight management? A big reason is that while it is easy to eat less in the short term, it is very hard to eat less for the rest of your life. Is there an alternative to focusing primarily on food intake? Yes, and it's really pretty simple.

To lose weight successfully you need to reduce the energy you consume in relation to the energy your body burns through your resting metabolism and your physical activity. This is not new—most weight management plans work on this principle. What's new is that the Step Diet does not focus on counting calories or eating particular foods like other plans. Instead, the Step Diet focuses on steps. That's right, steps, but in this case, three kinds of steps: BodySteps, LifeSteps, and MegaSteps.

It's really very simple. Diets that focus on calories or carbohydrate or fat grams are difficult. Think about yesterday. How many calories do you think you consumed? How many did your body burn in physical activity? If you are like most people, you have no idea.

Steps, on the other hand, can be easily measured with the step counter that comes with this book. All you have to do is wear it. It will count the number of steps you take each day very accurately. And since your resting metabolism can also be measured in steps (we'll show you how in Chapter 4), this means you can keep track of the total energy your body burns—in steps. Even more exciting is that we're going to show you how to convert the energy (in other words, the calories) in food into steps. Once you know how to do that, you'll be able to monitor your personal energy balance in steps: how much you've eaten in steps; how much energy your body burns in steps. Once you think of your energy balance in steps, you can approach weight loss logically. As you lose weight, your metabolism goes down. This is because your body is getting smaller and requires less energy. It happens to everyone who loses weight, and there is just no way to prevent it. And it is the reason that most people fail at keeping weight off. Because your metabolism has dropped, you have to eat substantially fewer calories than you did before weight loss in order to stay at your new, lower weight. In other words, you have to eat less—forever. It is almost impossible for most people to do that for a long time, so the weight comes back.

The Step Diet works for long-term weight management because it shows you how to increase the number of steps you take each day to compensate for the drop in your metabolism. As the amount of energy your resting metabolism burns gradually drops, the number of steps you walk gradually increases, so that the total amount of energy your body burns will be similar after weight loss to what it was before weight loss. When you have finished losing weight with the Step Diet, you will be able to eat much more food than you would have been able to eat with other diets because your total daily energy expenditure will be higher. Now you will have a real chance to keep that weight off forever.

The Five Principles of the Step Diet

In the Step Diet, we bring the latest scientific knowledge about weight loss and maintenance of weight loss to you. Much of this research has been done with people who have successfully lost weight and kept it off long term. From this research, we have developed five principles for successful weight management:

principle 1   **Maintain the proper energy balance.** Your weight is a direct consequence of the relationship between your energy intake and your energy expenditure. If you take in more energy than you burn (regardless of what kind of food you eat), you will gain weight. If you burn more energy than you take in, you will lose weight. Maintaining a constant weight, no matter what that weight is, requires you to balance the energy in the food you eat with the energy you burn. *The Step Diet provides you with the simple tools you need to manage your personal energy balance.*

principle 2   **Small changes drive success.** You have probably tried to make big lifestyle changes before—no carbs, no sugar, all liquids, whatever—and you have probably discovered that what is possible for weeks or even months becomes impossible over time. Consequently, you have lost and gained, lost and gained. *With the Step Diet, you can break that devastating (and unhealthy) cycle by learning to make small, sustainable changes in how much energy your body burns and how much energy you take in.*

principle 3   **Start with physical activity.** A major focus of the Step Diet is on physical activity. This is because your body is designed to work best when you are physically active. A key reason why people cannot keep weight off is that they are not prepared to increase their physical activity permanently. Once you go off your diet, it stands to reason that you will put pounds back on if you start taking in more energy in the food you eat without increasing your physical activity. The good news is that you don't have to sign up for the New York City Marathon to burn more energy—*with the Step Diet, all you have to do is walk more each day.*

principle 4 **Anticipate success, but not instantly.** It will take time for you to see the results of the Step Diet, but it will be time well spent. By starting with small, incremental changes in how you eat and how much you move—and accepting that your goal is long-term weight management rather than a quick fix— *you'll find yourself building the confidence you need to stay on course to your weight-loss goal.*

principle 5 **The maintenance of weight loss is more important than the speed or amount of weight loss.** Most people want to lose weight as quickly as possible, which isn't that hard to do. The hard part is keeping the weight off. The Step Diet shows you how to lose weight *and* keep it off—without feeling constantly deprived of food. *With the Step Diet, you will learn to keep some weight off before you lose more. It may take longer than some other diets to work, but the results will last.*

The Six Stages of Weight Control

The best way to approach a big project is to break it down into small, manageable pieces. Permanent weight management is a very big project, so we have broken it down into six stages:

stage 1 (seven days): **Prepare for permanent weight management.** You need to know what you are eating and how much physical activity you are currently getting in order to know what to change. Taking time at the beginning to determine this will pay off later.

stage 2 (two weeks): **Stop gaining weight.** You need to complete this stage even if you are not actively gaining weight now. Why? Because before you can learn to lose weight, you have to learn what makes you gain it. And it isn't just eating too much that keeps adding the pounds. The changes you make to stop gaining weight will lay the foundation both for losing weight and for keeping it off.

stage 3 (time it takes you to read Chapter 4): **Set your personal weight-management goals.** Here you'll learn to give yourself a personal weight-management target to shoot for that is realistic and sound for you. You'll also learn how to track your progress toward that goal. Equipped with only your bathroom scale, your step counter, and a food record, you will be well on your way to weight management.

stage 4 (twelve weeks maximum): **Make small changes to lose weight.** This is the core weight loss period during which you will make small changes in how much you eat and how many steps you take each day. You can expect to lose 1 to 2 pounds each week— exactly the rate that maximizes your chances of keeping the weight off.

stage 5 **(four weeks minimum): Find your personal energy balance point.** This crucial stage is where you learn how to keep your weight off. It calls for a different approach than you used when losing weight. During this stage, you devise a personal strategy for balancing the energy you eat with the energy your body burns—a strategy that fits comfortably into your lifestyle. You will learn how to use steps, not calories, to maintain energy balance. Even if you want to lose more weight, you must first believe that you can maintain your previous weight loss.

stage 6 **(as long as it takes): Plan for lifelong success.** Think of this stage as your graduate seminar. Here you'll learn some simple, fun ways to refine your energy balance skills. Most important, you'll learn how to make weight management a habit in your life, something you no longer have to think about all the time—you'll just do it!

When you've finished Stages 5 and 6, you may be ready to lose even more weight. Simply reset your goal (Stage 3) and repeat Stages 4 through 6. You can do this as many times as you like before you decide that you cannot make and sustain any further behavior changes. Notice that you are in charge. You decide on a weight loss you can maintain. You build in success up front. And you avoid the frustration that comes with losing more weight than you can comfortably keep off.

Whether you want to lose and keep off 10 pounds or 50, it is important to complete all six stages of the Step Diet. Obviously, a person who wants to lose and keep off 50 pounds will have to make greater lifestyle changes. Likewise, the time and effort required to accomplish each of the six stages will also vary from person to person. None of that matters now. Just start from where you are at this moment and get ready to make small but meaningful changes in your diet and physical activity

Success Story 1
Pounds on the Rebound

Jill hardly ever stepped on her bathroom scale, but each time she did, she was a bit heavier than before. And those "bits" added up over time—until eighteen years after graduating from college, the scale informed her that she had added 40 pounds since receiving her diploma! So Jill went on a high-fat, high-protein, low-carbohydrate regimen—and proceeded to shed all her postgraduate baggage in just a few weeks. Unfortunately, her excess weight just went on sabbatical—a year later, it was all back, plus 5 pounds more.

Problem: This diet provided Jill with a way to lose weight but not a way to live her life that would keep the weight off.

Solution: The Step Diet. Though at first Jill was frustrated at losing only 1 or 2 pounds a week, she found it easy to make small changes in the way she ate and exercised. She didn't feel excessively hungry eating a little less, and she got into the habit of taking a fifteen-minute walk before work—which had the added bonus of making her feel more alert and giving her a jump start on the day.

Most important, the Step Diet helped Jill feel in control of her weight. She lost 22 pounds in twelve weeks. Though she had wanted to lose 45 pounds, she realized it was not realistic to expect such a dramatic change without having the right follow-up plan. Jill is no longer the victim of yo-yo dieting—and she now feels she has the control to sustain whatever weight loss she achieves.

patterns. These changes may be so small as to be hardly noticeable. But the difference they'll make in the end will be enormous.

How to Use This Book

You might read *The Step Diet Book* straight through and then decide whether you want to try it. Or you might progress through it a section at a time as you follow the diet. Either way is okay. But we urge you to follow each of the six stages in order. You may be tempted to skip stages, but your chances of success multiply the more closely you follow the program.

We have included a lot of charts and tables in this book. We will ask you to make several calculations using these charts and tables. This is necessary in order to personalize your weight management. We want you to understand that your energy balance is different from other people's energy balance. You can fill in the charts and make the calculations right in the book, or you can make copies of those pages. But whatever you do, start now. The time and effort it takes will be worth it.

CHAPTER 1

Setting the Stage for Success

STAGE 1:
Prepare for permanent weight management.

Keep track of how much you eat and how much you move for seven days.

Y ou probably already realize that you are not as physically active as you would like to be, and that you are eating too much as well. You probably *don't* know, though, exactly how much exercise you're getting or how many calories you're taking in.

Your job over the next seven days is to pay close attention to your current eating and physical activity patterns *without changing them*. You have to know what you are doing now before you can begin to change, and you have to be able to live with the changes you make.

How to Wear and Use Your Step Counter

- Wear the step counter on your waistband or belt 2 to 6 inches on either side of your belly button.

- Make sure it is straight and close to your body.

- For women wearing clothes without a belt or waistband, try wearing the step counter on your undergarments or in the center of your bra. (The counter measures changes in your body's center of gravity.)

- If you have a large stomach, try placing the step counter on the side of your hip.

- To check that the step counter is working properly, put it on and count while you walk 100 steps. Your step counter should register between 90 and 110. If not, readjust it (by moving it closer to or farther from your belly button) and check it again.

- Wear your step counter all day, except when bathing or swimming (it is not waterproof). Most people get the majority of their steps through regular daily activities.

- Take off your step counter when you go to bed, and record your steps in a daily log book (see opposite page).

- Step counters will not register activities such as cycling, swimming, or weight lifting. You can convert these and other activities into their step equivalents, however, by using the chart on pages 98–99.

Take the First Step

Clip the step counter that came with this book onto your waistband or belt. It will give you, probably for the first time, an accurate measure of how much you move during the day. Put it on when you get up and wear it all the time (except when showering and sleeping). In other words, think of the step counter as an article of clothing.

Since your goal for weight loss and keeping weight off will be not in calories but in steps, we want you to get used to thinking in terms of steps rather than calories. But before you can develop specific goals for increasing steps that make sense for you, you need to know how many steps you take in a typical day right now.

SUCCESS TIP

Don't try to increase your physical activity during the seven-day preparation period. This week is for determining your baselines for eating and energy expenditure. If you "cheat," you won't get an accurate read on how you need to increase your daily calorie burning.

DAY	NUMBER OF STEPS
SUNDAY	
MONDAY	
TUESDAY	
WEDNESDAY	
THURSDAY	
FRIDAY	
SATURDAY	
Weekly Total	
Daily Average	

How to Determine Your Usual Number of Steps

1. Start on any day of the week and write down the number of steps you take each day for the next seven days. Write down your step number before you go to bed, then reset your step counter for the next day.

2. Add the total number of steps you have for the seven days. This is your weekly total. Divide this number by 7 to get your daily average.

AVERAGE NUMBER OF STEPS PER DAY BY AGE

Males

13–15	6,749
16–17	8,283
18–29	6,382
30–39	5,819
40–49	6,312
50–59	5,703
60+	4,515

Females

13–15	8,130
16–17	6,256
18–29	5,318
30–39	5,162
40–49	5,780
50–59	4,537
60+	4,504

Are You "In Step" or "Out of Step" with the General Population?

We designed and carried out a research study with Harris Polls to see how many steps Americans take. One thousand people were asked to wear step counters for two days (see the results in the tables to the left). In general, women report about 500 fewer steps a day than men. Not surprisingly, those who are overweight reported about 1,500 to 2,000 fewer steps a day than those who are not overweight. Since health authorities believe that most people should be getting 10,000 steps or more per day (and children even more), this survey shows that Americans are simply not moving enough. This is cause for real concern.

Pay Attention to Your Eating Patterns

Most people overeat on a regular basis without even realizing it, a habit we call passive overeating. It means eating when you are not really hungry or continuing to eat when you are already full. If you take a second helping of mashed potatoes when your meal has already filled you, you have engaged in passive overeating. If you find that you have eaten a whole bag of potato chips when you were not that hungry, you have engaged in passive overeating. We all do it. Eating whenever food is available is part of our genetic code—we need to eat to stay alive—and in today's world, food is always available. And for many of us, food has the added benefit of making us feel better, if only

Q. **I am traveling this week, so would it be better to wait until next week to start Stage 1?**

A. **If you travel frequently, this week may be more typical than you think, and you should go ahead and set your baseline for steps and food intake. If you rarely travel, wait until next week to start.**

temporarily. Still, whatever your reason for overeating—habit, availability, boredom, stress, or depression—it is important for you to understand passive overeating so that you can stop it. Here's how.

We want you to write down all the foods and beverages you consume over the next seven days and make a note of those times when you overate—meaning that you ate when you were not really hungry, continued to eat after you were full, or ate too much because of stress or other emotions. Don't forget that muffin you ate with your morning coffee, the handful of M&M's you munched while watching TV, *everything*. At this stage, you do not need to change what you eat. Just monitor it. Be honest—no one but you will see what you write down.

Most people don't like keeping a food record. However, it is only for a week and it is essential for your long-term success. (For some people, just writing down what they eat rduces their passive overeating.) Think of it as investing a few minutes each day for a week that will pay off continuously for the rest of your life.

How Much Is Too Much?

You'll find it easier to keep track of how much you eat if you know how much you usually serve in your bowls, coffee mugs, and

SUCCESS TIP

K eep track of *when* during the day you eat your meals and snacks. This will help you pinpoint problem times that need the most attention when you begin to take more control of your daily intake.

glasses. This first week, using a measuring cup and spoons, figure out what an average serving means in your home. Then use the following list to measure the foods you typically eat; adjust the items to match your usual foods. When you write down a serving size, be sure to measure food *after* it is cooked.

Once you've established your personal serving sizes, you may want to see how they measure up to recommended portion sizes. By simply using your hand, you can begin to visualize the difference between what *you* eat and what nutritionists have in mind when they list a typical serving size on a food label. Getting in touch with what a healthy portion looks like will pay big dividends as you gain control over your weight and build skills for lifelong weight management.

FOOD	USUAL AMOUNT YOU EAT
EXAMPLE: MILK	8 OUNCES
MILK	
CEREAL	
CHEESE	
LUNCH MEAT	
PASTA	
RICE	
BEEF	
CHICKEN	
FISH	
BUTTER	
MARGARINE	
SOUR CREAM	
SALAD DRESSING	
PEANUT BUTTER	
MAYONNAISE	
WINE	
BEER	
SODA	
ICE CREAM	
COOKIES	
POTATO CHIPS	

- 1 fist = 1 cup of cereal, pasta, or vegetables
- 1 finger = 1 ounce of cheese
- 1 thumb tip = 1 teaspoon of peanut butter, butter, or sugar
- 1 palm = 3 ounces of meat, fish, or poultry
- 1 handful = 1 ounce of nuts, chips, or pretzels

Here are some other objects you can use to estimate portion size:

- 1 hockey puck = $1/2$ cup
- 1 tennis ball = 1 medium fruit serving
- 1 deck of cards = 3 ounces of cooked meat
- 1 Ping-Pong ball = 2 tablespoons of butter, salad dressing, or peanut butter

The Food Record

There's no simple device like a step counter that can measure your food intake, but you need to get a handle on your eating habits. That's why we want you to fill in a food record each day for one week. In the first column, specify whether you were eating a meal or a snack. In the second column, write the time of day. Record the foods eaten in the third column and the amounts in the fourth column. In the last column, record whether you overate at that eating episode (consider the whole eating episode). Record yes if:

- You ate when you were not really hungry.
- You continued eating after you were full.
- You felt "too full" after eating.
- You ate too much as a reaction to stress, depression, or another emotion.

Q: My husband and I have been using our hands to estimate portion sizes, but my fist is much smaller than his. Is he eating too much, or am I eating too little?

A: Determining portion sizes with your fist is a convenient approximation—that is, it's not 100 percent accurate, but close enough. Besides, your husband's larger fist probably means he is bigger than you are, which also means that he requires more energy each day.

Once you become aware of your overeating, it will be much easier for you to stop doing it. Indeed, you may start to lose weight even before you begin the Step Diet, which will be powerful reinforcement.

Notice that we are not asking you to calculate the number of calories you eat. This is because counting calories is hard, takes too much time, and isn't necessary for you to succeed in weight management. Studies from the University of Wisconsin have clearly shown that people underestimate the number of calories they eat by several hundred calories per day. It's just too hard to accurately remember all of the food you eat.

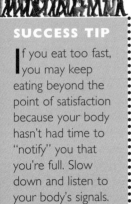

SUCCESS TIP

If you eat too fast, you may keep eating beyond the point of satisfaction because your body hasn't had time to "notify" you that you're full. Slow down and listen to your body's signals.

We think it is ironic that most weight-loss plans rely on having you count calories when it is so hard to do accurately. Sure, it does help to get you focused on what you eat, but there are easier ways to do this, such as focusing on when you overeat. We want you to keep food records not to count calories, but to increase your awareness of when and how often you eat more than you really want or how often you eat when you are not really hungry.

You will have learned so much about your eating patterns by the end of this week! And you're probably raring to go on the weight-loss portion of this program. But patience. First you have to tackle the biggest thorn in the dieter's side: the tendency to gain back the weight we lose.

SEVEN-DAY FOOD RECORD EXAMPLE — Day 1

Eating Occasion	Time of Day	Food	Amount	Overeating
Breakfast	6:45 A.M.	Cheerios cereal	1 fistful (1 cup)	No
		2 percent milk	1 cup	
		Coffee with	2 mugs	
		cream and sugar	(3 cups) coffee,	
			1 tablespoon	
			cream,	
			1 teaspoon	
			sugar each	
Snack	10:00 A.M.	Energy bar	2-ounce bar	No
Lunch	12:30 P.M.	McDonald's	1	Yes
		double		
		cheeseburger		
		French fries	Large	
		Coke	(32 ounces)	
Snack	3:00 P.M.	Apple	1 medium	No
		Water	2 8-ounce glasses	
Dinner	6:30 P.M.	Tossed salad with	1 cup salad,	Yes
		ranch dressing	2 tablespoons	
			dressing	
		Spaghetti with	3 fistfuls	
		tomato sauce	(3 cups)	
		French bread	2 slices with	
		with margarine	1 tablespoon	
			margarine	
		Red wine	1 glass (6 ounces)	
		Chocolate ice	1 bowl (1 1/2 cups)	
		cream		

SEVEN-DAY FOOD RECORD				Day 1
Eating Occasion	Time of Day	Food	Amount	Overeating

SEVEN-DAY FOOD RECORD				Day 2
Eating Occasion	Time of Day	Food	Amount	Overeating

SEVEN-DAY FOOD RECORD				Day 3
Eating Occasion	Time of Day	Food	Amount	Overeating

SEVEN-DAY FOOD RECORD				Day 4
Eating Occasion	Time of Day	Food	Amount	Overeating

SEVEN-DAY FOOD RECORD				Day 5
Eating Occasion	**Time of Day**	**Food**	**Amount**	**Overeating**

SEVEN-DAY FOOD RECORD				Day 6
Eating Occasion	Time of Day	Food	Amount	Overeating

SEVEN-DAY FOOD RECORD				Day 7
Eating Occasion	Time of Day	Food	Amount	Overeating

CHAPTER 2

Why Do We Gain It Back?

In this chapter, you will begin your education about weight management. It's an easy course with no homework, no grades, and absolutely no lectures, but it is an essential prerequisite for everything that will come later.

Let's start with the creeping weight gain we talked about earlier, that 1 to 2 pounds a year that most of us add on. It may surprise you to learn that most of this excess weight comes from fewer than 100 extra calories each day. That's right, just 100 calories per day—fewer than the number of calories in a can of soda or a candy bar—are the chief cause of our alarming trend toward obesity.

THE 100-CALORIE CLUB

How to tack on an extra 100 calories during the day:

- Supersize your french fries
- Eat an extra ¹/₂ bagel
- Drink an extra soft drink
- Add an extra tablespoon of salad dressing

Here's how it works: Your body converts excess calories (more than are burned by your metabolism and your physical activity) to energy that is stored in the body (mostly as fat). Since your body is not 100 percent efficient, it does not convert all the extra calories to body fat; some are burned in the conversion process. If we assume that your body is 50 percent efficient at this process (most people are probably more efficient than this), half of all your excess calories would be converted to energy stored in your body. Therefore, if you eat 100 more calories than you burn each day, you would be storing half (50 calories per day). Over a year, you would add 18,250 calories of stored energy to your body. You gain 1 pound of weight for each 3,500 calories you store in your body. This would equal a 5-pound gain in body weight over a year. You could gain 2 pounds each year from just an extra 40 calories each day.

We Have a "Growing" Crisis

In the United States, about 65 percent of the population is considered overweight. And the rest of the world is rapidly catching up. In fact, average body weight is gradually increasing in almost every country in the world. Using our analysis of large population surveys, we predict that 75 percent of U.S. adults will be overweight by the year 2008 unless something is done to reverse the trend.

This increase in obesity is not due to anything in the water. Nor is it simply due to people eating the wrong kinds of foods—too many fats, too many carbs, too much sugar. It is due to too many people getting more energy in the foods they eat than they burn each day. It is about energy balance. Here are the basics of energy balance:

> **WEIGHT AND SEE**
>
> Some obesity experts predict we could all be overweight by 2050!

- When **energy intake = energy burned,** you are in *energy balance.*
- When **energy intake is greater than energy burned,** you are in *positive energy balance* and gaining weight.
- When **energy intake is less than energy burned,** you are in *negative energy balance* and losing weight.

You have gained extra weight because you have been in positive energy balance—you got more energy in the food you ate than you burned, and your body stored the excess energy, primarily as body fat. Your weight problems are not going to be permanently solved by avoiding carbs, fats, sugar, or any other types of foods. In fact, you have probably avoided all of these at some time in your life. Sure, these strategies work in the short term because by focusing on avoiding something (anything), you will eat less. They don't work in the long term because they are not addressing the real problem.

If you are taking in the same amount of energy as you burn each day, you will not gain weight. It doesn't matter if you eat all carbs or all fats or all sugars or all Twinkies (though we wouldn't recommend this!). You won't gain weight. Your weight can change only when you are not in energy balance: when the energy in the food you eat is not the same as the energy you burn. This is the essence of the Step Diet. If you want to lose weight, burn more energy than you take in. Regardless of what you eat, you will lose weight. But you can't stop there; no one can lose weight forever. To keep your weight off permanently, you must reach a new

SUCCESS TIP

Almost all of us underestimate how much we eat. For example, would you have guessed that the average pasta serving in a restaurant is *6 cups?* This is two to three times more than a healthy serving. We are living in a "super-sized" environment, and our sense of what a reasonable portion size looks like has become skewed by servings outside the home, like the enormous soda and popcorn containers offered in movie theaters. Reeducate yourself as to what a healthy portion of food looks like.

state of energy balance where the energy you take in is equal to the energy you burn, but at a smaller body weight.

So why do so many of us today have trouble keeping extra weight off? This was not a problem that plagued our grandparents and great-grandparents. The answer is all around us. No matter where you go—your home, your work, bookstores, gas stations—there's food. Plentiful, yummy, inexpensive food. Remember, humans have evolved to guard against starvation. Our genes tell us to eat whenever food is available—and in today's environment, food is always available. In addition, the portions of food we get in restaurants and serve at home have increased substantially over the years. And research from Dr. Barbara Rolls at Penn State University has shown that the more food there is on the plate, the more we tend to eat. This is a perfect example of passive overeating. We aren't that hungry, but we can't pass up a good deal.

No wonder we're gaining weight! Check out the chart on the next page to see the boost in portion sizes over the past quarter century if you're not convinced.

At the same time, most people no longer need to be physically active to find food and shelter and provide basic needs for their families. Actually, it's quite the opposite. And the more labor-saving devices we rely on, the more calories we conserve. For instance, just by using elevators and escalators rather than stairs, the average woman can build up a reserve of 4,160 calories a year. This could translate into a $1^1/_2$-pound weight gain. And a man who relies on his remote to change TV channels might store 819

PORTION DISTORTION			
Food	1977 Portion Size	Current Portion Size	Percent of Caloric Increase
Hamburger (average size)	5.7 ounces	7 ounces	23 percent
Soft drinks	13 ounces	20 ounces	54 percent
Mexican combination plate	6.3 ounces	8 ounces	27 percent
Snack foods (potato chips, pretzels, crackers, etc.)	1 ounce	1.6 ounces	60 percent
Bagel	2 ounces	4 ounces	100 percent
French fries	3.1 ounces	3.6 ounces	16 percent

calories a year that he could be burning if he got up off his duff. This doesn't sound like much, but it can add 1/4 pound of body fat.

The way we spend our leisure time is also a factor in weight gain. Most of us have more leisure time than ever before, but we don't seem to be spending it being physically active. Is this any surprise given the attraction of hundreds of channels of television, DVDs, video games, computers? We spend our leisure time being sedentary, and we are not likely to get any more active as technology brings us better and better sedentary entertainment.

Why More and More Children Are Overweight

It should come as no surprise that even our kids are overweight. After all, they are exposed to the same influences as our increasingly heavy adult population. In addition, children are less well equipped to resist or

Success Story 2

"Benched" Athlete Enters New Arena of Activity

Fred is a great example of how the environment can contribute to a weight problem. During his early adult years, he regularly played basketball with his buddies and rarely ate out except for special occasions. But as he became more successful in his insurance career, he no longer had time to shoot hoops, and he ate out just about every day as part of business meetings and travel. Over the next decade, the basketball he no longer dribbled downcourt took up residence under his shirt—he gained 30 pounds!

After starting the Step Diet, Fred learned other ways to build regular physical activity into his day and reduce the amount of food he was eating. He still didn't have time to play basketball, but there was always time to walk. He began to park in the far end of the company lot, which added 1,000 steps per day. He started emptying wastebaskets in his house every day. On days when he didn't have business lunches, he'd bring a light lunch from home and walk from his office to local stores to do errands, instead of driving as he used to. Fred didn't lose all of his 30 pounds (he lost 10), but he stopped his gradual weight gain *and* improved his health.

cope with the influences that foster obesity in today's world. At least adults can use their knowledge, skills, and financial means to help overcome the constant pressure of an environment that promotes weight gain.

Our children are exposed at an early age to both old and modern cultural norms that promote excess energy intake and low energy expenditure. Consider the time-honored practice of telling kids to "clean your plate." Research conducted by Dr. Leann Birch at Penn State University has demonstrated repeatedly that this practice is counterproductive in kids because it undermines their ability to recognize when they are full. It is also common for parents to reward good behavior with special treats, such as candy and desserts. A child learns very early that she can manipulate the situation to gain access to the treat, whether or not she has consumed a well-balanced meal with lots of nutrients. Of course, parents past and present have always had the best intentions in mind when feeding their children. For centuries, our grandmothers have instilled in us the notion that "food is love"—and who doesn't want all the love they can get?

Enter modern cultural norms. More and more families have two working parents. This means we have less time to prepare and eat family meals together at home, and to make sure our children are staying active so they can burn up that excess energy they're taking in. We eat out more, and the food we eat outside the home is typically higher in fat and calories. Overlarge portions cause our kids to passively overeat, just like adults do. And fast food has invaded even our schools, where vending machines with high-calorie snacks and beverages are now commonplace. Though there may be healthier choices for kids in these locations, without a parent supervising them, how many kids are going to choose an apple over a bag of chocolate chip cookies?

Too often we may use television and video games as baby-sitters so we can get things done around the house. With suburban sprawl, fewer kids can walk or bike to school, and fears for their safety often keep them from playing outside much. They stay indoors safe and sound—and sedentary. The unintended consequence of all these features of contemporary life is that kids' physical fitness levels are at an all-time low. How can we expect their bodies to keep them at a normal weight with all these forces working against them?

Meanwhile, the home front is hardly a health spa. High-fat microwaveable foods filling the freezer, a hundred TV channels to surf through, video games that turn kids into motionless robots—all of these modern home "conveniences" conspire against the healthy eating and activity that would provide an optimum energy balance among today's youth.

> ### LIFETIME MEMBERSHIP IN THE CLEAN PLATE CLUB
>
> Telling kids to finish every morsel at mealtime can make them unable to accurately perceive when they are full—and the inability persists into adulthood.

What's the solution to a situation that sounds so hopeless? First of all, parents must get involved. It is up to them to instill healthy habits in their children early in life, by what they say and what they do, and then support and reinforce these habits on a daily basis. And while it is difficult to face a situation in which a child might be gaining excessive weight, taking the right action with your child can help chart a new course away from weight problems—and toward a healthier, more active adulthood with a lower risk of health problems. Second, realize that while you might not be able to change everything at once, small changes can have a big impact.

Push Back Against the Environment

Our bodies have strong defenses against losing weight, which means we have very few defenses against gaining it. This is not surprising, because at one time it was an advantage to have extra energy stored as body fat. Our ancestors had to be very physically active and often faced food shortages, so having a reserve could be essential for survival during lean times. Clearly, this is irrelevant for most people in our modern world of vast supermarkets and high technology. The point is, you can't count on your body to take care of your weight, because it still sees fat as an asset.

However, it *is* possible to resist the push of the environment toward weight gain and keep from being in positive energy balance. Doing this takes brainpower, not just willpower. Many strong-willed people gain weight because they have not learned to use their brain to help manage their weight. Successful weight loss is about having the knowledge and skills you need to take an active role in managing your weight. It is about understanding how to maximize your body's weight-regulation systems so you're in control. It is about deciding you don't want to keep adding 10 to 20 pounds every decade. This is not going to happen if you don't make it happen—every day.

Let's say you're on a diet to lose weight. You get down to a desired level. Then you stop dieting, because you don't want to lose any more weight—and because you can't endure the rigors of the diet any longer. So there you are, at the weight you want—but not for long. Since you're not dieting anymore, you start taking in more energy. What does this do? The extra calories announce themselves on your bathroom scale! Before you know it, you're right back to square one.

Small Changes Drive Success

The key to successful weight loss is pretty straightforward: You have to keep your weight from getting worse before you can begin to make it better. We are going to show you how to do this by making progressive small changes to your lifestyle. Typically messages from health professionals advocate big lifestyle changes, such as totally changing the kinds of foods you eat or joining a health club or gym. The problem with big lifestyle changes is that most people cannot sustain them. By making small changes, you set yourself up for long-term success. You feel good when you achieve one goal and are motivated to go to the next one. You have a better chance of making permanent lifestyle changes when you make these changes gradually.

The Quick Fix

Most popular weight-loss programs do not take the time to teach you about energy balance. These programs focus on a quick fix, because that is what the program developers think you want. And history seems to prove them right. If you look at the best-selling diet books over the past twenty years, most focus on losing weight quickly. They do this by finding a gimmick for you to focus on—avoiding carbs, avoiding fats, eating grapefruits, or drinking beer. You lose weight because you eat less. You just don't *keep* it off. If any of these diets worked, why would we have so many different diet books?

Furthermore, these diets give little attention to physical activity. The more you limit your food intake, the greater your state of negative energy balance, and the more weight you lose. But your metabolic rate also goes down with big reductions in energy intake, and it stays down because you are losing body mass. As your metabolic rate goes down, your body burns less energy. Because your body is now burning less

TURNING FAT INTO PROFIT

Americans spend over $100 billion per year on weight-loss products and services.

energy, your energy balance becomes less negative, and your weight loss slows dramatically. You get frustrated because you are very hungry, yet you are not losing weight as fast as you were initially. Finally, you get tired of being hungry all the time and go back to eating the way you did before. Because your metabolic rate has declined, your increased food intake puts you in very positive energy balance, and you regain all of your weight very quickly. Sound familiar?

If you have struggled with your weight for a while, you know that the quick fixes are not likely to work. The problem is that you have never before had a reasonable alternative. The Step Diet is not the easy, quick method to weight loss but the successful, long-term method. It involves taking the time to learn why you are gaining weight and to learn some basic energy balance skills that allow you to set and achieve your individual weight-loss goals. It is not going to happen quickly. But you can be successful; thousands of people have been.

SUCCESS TIP

If you are able to change your lifestyle only temporarily, you will be able to change your weight only temporarily. If you want to change your weight permanently, you will have to change your lifestyle permanently.

Q: **What if I don't like to exercise?**

A: **You don't have to join a gym or wear spandex to succeed at the Step Diet. You just add steps to your day. We will give you tips throughout the book to help you increase your movement each day, and your step counter will give you "real time" feedback on how well you are accomplishing this goal.**

You've Got to Have a Plan

Imagine a carpenter starting out to build a house by going to the store and buying some lumber, a hammer, and nails. Sure, he could build something, but without a plan, it isn't likely his structure would be something you'd want to live in. The same holds true for weight management. If you start by simply eating less, you will probably lose some weight. But you will be dissatisfied with the long-term result, just as you would be with a house that was thrown together without a plan and without your needs in mind.

If you have lost weight and kept it off for more than one or two years, you are a rare individual. While millions of people lose weight, only 5 to 20 percent (no one knows the exact number) keep it off. If your goal is merely to be one of the millions who lose weight, you can choose any

Success Story 3

Escaping the Trap of "Do-or-Die" Diets

Melissa picked up a popular diet book at her local bookstore. She followed the plan rigorously for the first three weeks and lost some weight. But the diet plan was so restrictive that Melissa had a difficult time following it when she wanted to eat at a restaurant or at a friend's house. When she strayed from the diet's rigid plan, she felt she had to virtually starve herself the next day to "catch up." Within a month, Melissa had stopped following the plan and had regained her weight.

Finally, Melissa decided to try the Step Diet and make small, sustainable changes to lose weight and keep it off. Melissa found that by walking more each day and reducing her portion sizes, she was able to lose weight and, more important, maintain the loss over time.

diet book in the bookstore. If you want to be one of those few who really succeed in weight management, you need the complete plan that the Step Diet gives you.

The first and most important lifestyle change you will make on the Step Diet is to increase your physical activity. No diet anywhere will allow you to maintain a healthy weight with the low levels of physical activity that most people get. Here is what science tells us: If physical activity is low, the total energy your body burns will also be low. In this condition, you can avoid gaining weight only by constantly restricting the calories in the food you eat. You can do this for only so long. When you relax your vigilance, you gain weight.

Scientific research conducted by us, as well as studies from researchers at Harvard and the Cooper Institute, shows that two things happen when you increase your physical activity. First, you can eat more food without being in positive energy balance, and, second, your body becomes better at regulating your appetite. If you were able to increase your physical activity enough (say, to the level of physical activity that was common in your great-grandparents' day), you would not likely have to worry much about what you eat. This is impractical for most people in today's high-tech world. If you increase your physical activity modestly, you will still need to pay attention to how much you eat, but now your body's physiology is working for you. The increased activity helps your body work the way it was designed to work.

As an added bonus, physical activity improves your mood and enhances your overall quality of life. Once you get into a pattern of regular physical activity, you will feel better and will want to be more active—it is a positive feedback loop.

Remember—Small Changes Work

A big reason that many people fail at long-term weight management is because they try to make lifestyle changes that are too big. We bet most of you have tried this. It is natural to want to change as quickly as possible, but scientific research, including a review by the National Institutes of Health, and research from our laboratory, has shown over and over that few people can maintain large lifestyle changes. The science says that small changes can be sustainable, and the Step Diet leads you through the process of making small lifestyle changes.

Learning from the Masters

Thousands of individuals have used the techniques we suggest and have been remarkably successful in achieving permanent weight loss. They are members of the National Weight Control Registry (NWCR), a group established in 1994 by one of the authors of this book (Dr. James O. Hill) and Dr. Rena Wing, a behavioral psychologist at Brown University. More than fifteen scientific papers have been published describing how these individuals achieved long-term success in weight management. You will be hearing more about these people throughout this book, because much of what we know about successful long-term weight management comes from these "masters" of weight management. The more than 3,000 individuals in the NWCR have on average kept off 67 pounds for six years. Pretty impressive! There is only one thing NWCR members share in common about how they lost weight: More than 90 percent of them used *both* diet and physical activity. They dieted differently. They exercised differently. But whatever they did, they did both.

So can you.

CHAPTER 3

The 2,000-Step Difference

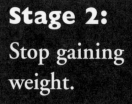

Stage 2: Stop gaining weight.

Walk 2,000 additional steps a day.

We'll let you in on a big secret. It's not really that hard to stop weight gain. In fact, you can stop gaining weight by making one small change to your current lifestyle. Just walk 2,000 more steps (about one mile) each day. You can do it all at once or spread it out during the day. It doesn't matter: You will burn an additional 100 calories, and it will take you all of fifteen or twenty minutes. Who can't find time for three 5-minute walks in a day?

Little Steps Mean a Lot

Many of you may be saying to yourselves, "I need to lose weight now. I can't be bothered guarding against a small yearly weight gain first." But remember that a key ingredient in the success of the Step Diet is understanding the power of small changes. What has happened in the past when you made the big, drastic lifestyle changes required by a new diet? Right. Do it differently this time, and you will not only lose weight but keep it off.

Consider a couple of analogies. First, let's say that you find yourself in serious debt. You are having trouble paying past bills and are accumulating new bills faster than you can keep up with them. A good strategy would be to consult a professional to show you how to take control of your finances. Your ultimate goal is to go from being in debt to accumulating money, but your financial adviser will no doubt tell you there is an important step in between, which you can't skip: *You must stop things from getting worse before you can learn how to make them better.* You have to stop getting further into debt before you can deal with your existing debt. In other words, first stabilize your situation, then work to improve it.

As another example, suppose you are in a car accident and have to go to the emergency room. The first goal of the ER staff is to stop the bleeding. Once you are stabilized and the medical staff is sure that things are not getting worse, they can develop a plan to help you begin healing.

Get the picture? First, you need to stabilize your weight (and your lifestyle) so your situation won't get worse (that is, so you are not gaining more weight). Only then can you follow through with the Step Diet and permanently fix your problem (lose weight and keep it off). Otherwise, you'll find yourself trapped in the typical weight gain/loss/gain cycle that sabotages so many well-laid plans.

THE 2,000-STEP DIFFERENCE

Success Story 4

One Small Step Leads to 12,000

During her seven-day preparation for the Step Diet, Donna found that she was eating pretty well, and her portions were not regularly out of control. She was stunned, however, at what she found out about her activity level. Donna, a stay-at-home mom who was continually shuttling her three young children from one place to another, considered herself an active person. After all, she was exhausted at the end of the day. But Donna had confused being busy with being active, and she was shocked to see that she was taking an average of only 4,500 steps a day.

With the revelation that she was spending so much time sitting in the car and being inactive, Donna found it easy to use her step counter to help her increase her steps. For example, by walking around the field instead of sitting to watch her children play baseball, soccer, and lacrosse, she easily increased her walking by 2,000 steps a day. Then she gave step counters to the other moms so that she could have company while she walked, and she added more and more steps to her routine. By the end of twelve weeks, she was regularly logging more than 12,000 steps a day!

Your First Small Change: Walk More

By now you have completed the seven-day preparation for weight loss and determined how many steps you take in a typical day. Your goal now is to walk 2,000 more steps each day than you did on an average day last week. If you are like most people, your number of steps varies from day to day, so it is important to determine the average number of steps you take each day. It doesn't matter how or when you get the extra steps, as long as your step counter reflects that you have made them.

But what is important is that you make 2,000 extra steps a permanent part of your daily routine. People tend to be creatures of habit, and we want you to get in the habit of walking a little more. Of course, it is okay if you exceed your 2,000-step goal on some days. At first, there may be days when you don't get your extra 2,000 steps, but keep trying

PUTTING STEPS IN A REAL-WORLD CONTEXT

The following estimates show you how far your steps take you. (Note: these are rough approximations; the actual number of steps will vary by individual and stride length.)

DISTANCE	NUMBER OF STEPS (2-FOOT STRIDE)	NUMBER OF STEPS (2.5-FOOT STRIDE)
FOOTBALL FIELD	150	120
QUARTER-MILE TRACK	660	528
MILE	2,640	2,112
CITY BLOCK ($1/20$ MILE)	132	106
EMPIRE STATE BUILDING (102 FLOORS)	1,860	

to meet this goal every day. In most cases, the more walking you do, the better, and it doesn't cost you anything. Remember, though, that the Step Diet is about small changes that can be maintained forever. If you try to increase your steps too quickly, you might get discouraged when you cannot maintain this level of walking.

While you are incorporating this extra walking into your day, you can read Chapter 4 and set your personal goals for weight management.

Success Story 5
Stepping It Up

During the seven days of preparing for permanent weight management with the Step Diet, Paul found he was walking about 6,000 steps a day—not bad. Still, he realized that in order to lose weight, he needed to squeeze in 2,000 more steps each day.

Paul began to have some fun figuring out how to fit in these extra steps. Here's how he did it:

- Parking in the farthest corner of his company parking lot = *500 extra steps*

- Walking up the stairs to his fifth-floor office = *500 extra steps*

- Walking down the hall to talk to co-workers instead of sending e-mails = *500 extra steps*

- Strolling up the street to get coffee instead of getting it in the basement cafeteria (to which he routinely took the elevator) = *500 extra steps*

- *Total extra daily steps = 2,000!*

Don't Forget the Feet!

Q: Yesterday I forgot to write down my steps and did not reset my step counter at the end of the day. What should I do?

A: Your step counter counts up to 99,999 steps. If you forget to record your step number and to reset your step counter one day, just divide the number at the end of the next day by 2.

A word of warning: without proper footwear, blisters, corns, and calluses can derail your efforts, so make sure you have a good pair of walking shoes. Here are some points to consider when making your selection:

• **Type of shoe.** Running shoes are fine, of course, but nowadays there are a number of shoes designed specifically for walking as well. We don't recommend cross-training shoes for high-volume walking, because they don't provide proper flexibility for the rolling motion of walking. A good walking shoe should have a life span of about 500 miles (about a million steps).

• **Fit.** Try on a wide variety of shoes to determine which one feels best, and be sure to try shoes on both feet (a person's feet are not always exactly the same size). Your heel should fit securely for good support, and the front of the shoe should be flexible so the foot rolls comfortably when you walk. Look for a high toe area so your toes won't be cramped.

• **Socks.** Consider buying specialized walking socks with extra padding along the bottom for long walks; they help prevent chafing and blisters. Socks made of some of

Q: My knees and hips start to ache when I walk for very long. Can I still follow the Step Diet if I prefer to get my physical activity in by swimming?

A: Absolutely! Any type of physical activity is encouraged in the Step Diet. Please see pages 98–99 for the step conversions for various types of swimming.

the new synthetic blends, rather than cotton, will draw perspiration away from the foot and increase your comfort.

Tips for Increasing Steps

At Work

- Take two ten-minute walks during the day.
- Choose the entrance to your building farthest from your parking spot.
- Host one "walking meeting" each day.
- Walk to a rest room, soda machine, or copy machine on a different floor.
- Walk a few laps around your floor during breaks.
- Walk to a colleague's office rather than sending an e-mail.
- Take five-minute walking breaks from your computer.
- Get off the bus earlier and walk the extra blocks to work.
- Take the stairs rather than the elevator or the escalator.
- Start a walking club with your co-workers.
- Walk while using a speaker or cordless phone.
- Get up and move at least once every thirty minutes.
- Find a lunch spot that is at least a ten-minute walk each way.
- Start a salsa dancing class at the lunch hour.

Add your own ideas below:

- _____
- _____

Q: I like to ride my bicycle. Does my step counter work during biking?

A. No. But the table on pages 98–99 will show you how to convert activities such as biking and swimming into steps that can be added to the number on your step counter.

Success Story 6

Leaving Pounds Back at the Office

Fran worked as a secretary for the president of a large corporation. She was usually at work early in the morning and often stayed to work overtime. Fran rarely left the building during her workday, and she always ate lunch at her desk. Most nights, she ate a microwave dinner, watched some television, and then went to bed. Not surprisingly, Fran found out that she typically took a mere 1,800 steps a day.

At first, Fran was so discouraged that she almost decided to abandon the Step Diet. If physical activity was essential for weight management, she figured she had no chance to be successful. But she decided to give it a try. She started going out to lunch with some of her co-workers. This usually added at least 1,000 steps to her day. She found that she could use the fax and copy machines on the floor below her and added another 500 daily steps. Finally, she found that she actually enjoyed planning a short walk around the block after she got home. She got in another 500 steps that way and got to know some of her neighbors better at the same time. When her boss, not exactly the picture of fitness himself, queried her about what she was doing, she gave him a step counter, too.

When Out and About

• Park farther away in store parking lots.

• Always return your grocery cart to the designated storage area.

• Avoid elevators and escalators—take the stairs.

• Walk—don't drive—for trips of less than one mile.

• Walk at the airport while waiting for your plane.

• Take several trips to unload your groceries from your car.

• Avoid drive-throughs—get out of your car and walk inside.

• Walk around the local flea market or mall.

• Go to the local museum.

• Attend a county fair.

• Walk to your nearest mailbox to mail a letter instead of leaving it for the mail carrier to pickup.

Q. How long do I need to wait before I can start losing weight?

A. This is really up to you. Once you are convinced that you can maintain the 2,000-step-per-day increase, you can move to the next phase of the Step Diet. For some people, this will be about two weeks. For others, it may be longer.

SAFETY TIPS WHEN WALKING

• Start at an easy pace.

• Carry identification with you.

• Carry a cell phone.

• Carry a bottle of water.

• Wear good shoes for walking.

• Wear sunscreen and a hat.

• Walk with a friend or tell someone the route you are taking.

• At night, carry a flashlight.

• Put reflectors on your shoes or wear reflective shoelaces.

- Listen to books on tape while you walk, and set yourself a goal: one chapter today, two tomorrow.
- Walk around the field or the gym at your kids' games.
- Pick up litter in your neighborhood or park.
- Visit a shut-in.
- Plant seeds.
- Form a walking group and meet at a set time each day.
- Take a walk in the rain.
- Try bird-watching or hiking.
- Window-shop—walk the mall before you buy.
- Visit the zoo—take a kid along.
- Take an historic walking tour of your city.
- Deliver neighborhood newsletters.
- Look for active volunteer opportunities.

Add your own ideas below:

- _____
- _____
- _____
- _____
- _____
- _____

Q. I have worn my step counter for a week now, and I am struggling to get in an extra 2,000 steps. I just don't have time. Can I still be successful with the Step Diet?

A. Those 2,000 steps sound like a lot, but in fact they equate to about fifteen to twenty minutes each day. If it seems overwhelming to get in the 2,000 steps all at once, add 500 steps this week (about five additional minutes of walking), then another 500 the next week, and see how you do.

At Home with Friends and Family

- Instead of reading the newspaper or watching the news on TV, put on your Walkman and listen to the news while you take a walk.
- Walk around your living room during TV commercials. (You can get close to 1,000 steps in a one-hour TV program.)

- Occasionally walk to the TV to change the channel.
- Take a "family walk" each evening and find your favorite routes.
- Go up and down the stairs with laundry or other household items separately instead of combining trips.
- Empty wastebaskets every day.
- Plan active vacations.
- Take advantage of nearby parks and hiking trails.
- Get your kids to take you for a walk.
- To make sure your kids move enough, make walking the dog their responsibility.
- Do a family challenge to see who can get the most steps.
- Reward kids/family members for meeting step goals.
- Walk to a neighbor's/friend's house instead of phoning.
- Play with your grandchildren in the park.
- Participate with the "Walking School Bus" program, where some neighborhood parents walk to school with neighborhood kids.
- Volunteer to be a school crossing guard.
- Rake the leaves in your neighbor's yard.
- Shovel the sidewalk in front of your neighbor's house.
- Learn the latest dance moves with your family.
- Spread a packet of wildflower seeds around an open field.

Add your own ideas below:

- _____
- _____
- _____
- _____
- _____
- _____
- _____
- _____

Do It Your Way

After you've made walking an additional 2,000 steps a day part of your regular routine, you'll soon discover your own "best" ways to meet your goal. Write down ten ways you personally can get an extra 2,000 steps into your day, and share the list with your friends and family. Nothing breeds walking success like companionship!

Top Ten Ways to Walk More

1. _____

2. _____

3. _____

4. _____

5. _____

6. _____

7. _____

8. _____

9. _____

10. _____

CHAPTER 4

Know What You Want

Most people set unreasonable goals for weight loss. Take Selma, for example. Selma has always been overweight. She was one of the heaviest girls in every grade all through school. She weighed 180 pounds when she graduated from high school and 205 pounds when she graduated from college. Now, at age forty, she weighs 220 pounds. If asked, Selma would tell you that her goal weight is 140 pounds. Is it realistic that Selma will lose 80 pounds, more than 30 percent of her current weight? Sure, some people *have* lost 80 pounds. But very few can change their lives enough to keep off this amount of weight.

Stage 3:
Set your personal weight-management goals.

Be sure your goals are realistic for your weight.

We are not saying that Selma can't be one of these rare individuals, but we would not recommend 80 pounds as an initial weight-loss goal. If this is her goal and she loses only 40 pounds, she will consider herself a failure. Selma needs to realize that losing 40 pounds is a great accomplishment and that losing this amount will improve her long-term health tremendously.

Long-term success in weight management is more likely if your initial goal is feasible. This does not mean you should set yourself an easy goal; you need to feel a sense of achievement when you reach it. Then, and only then, should you increase your weight-loss goal.

What is a realistic goal for Selma on the Step Diet? More important, what is a realistic goal for you? That's what this chapter will help you determine.

Long-term success in weight management is more likely if you consider the following questions:

- What is your reason for wanting to lose weight (or keep from gaining weight)?
- How much weight loss is feasible for you?
- Are you willing to do what it takes to lose weight and keep it off?
- How will you measure success with the Step Diet?

Why Do You Want to Lose Weight?

We want you to take a few minutes and think about why you want to lose weight (or if you don't need to lose weight, why you want to keep from gaining weight). Why are you beginning the Step Diet? People lose weight for many reasons. You might want to lose weight because you are worried about your health. You might already have an obesity-related disease or be at high risk for such a disease. You might want to lose weight just to feel better; to improve your quality of life. Losing weight can give you more energy and can help you feel better about yourself. Individuals in the National Weight Control Registry tell us that their quality of life is higher after weight loss than before. You might want to lose weight just to be able to do some simple things, like tying your shoes or going up and down steps, that you couldn't do before weight loss. You might want to lose weight just to look better. We also know (from lots of personal experience) that you might want to lose weight for a class reunion, wedding, or other special event. Finally, some of you may want to use the Step Diet just to improve the quality of your diet or to become more physically fit.

It doesn't particularly matter why you want to lose weight. All of the above are perfectly reasonable reasons to lose weight with the Step Diet. The important thing is that you know why you want to lose weight. Many times, your reasons for wanting to lose weight are linked to whether or not you are willing to do what it takes to succeed. We hope you will write down the reason or reasons why you want to lose weight. It will be helpful for you to go back and look at this periodically, particularly during those times when you are struggling to stay with your weight-loss plan or to maintain your personal energy balance point to keep your weight off.

I want to lose weight because:

1. _____

2. _____

3. _____

Your Body Mass Index

Your body mass index, or BMI, is a useful number for you to know, just like your cholesterol or blood pressure levels, which is why your physician should assess your BMI at your office visits. BMI provides information to you (and your physician) about the health risks of your body weight. BMI is calculated as weight (in kilograms) divided by height squared (in meters). The table on pages 48–49 converts kilograms and meters into pounds and inches. Simply find your height in the BMI table, then move to the right in that same row until you reach the column with your weight. For example, if you are 64 inches (5 feet, 4 inches) tall and weigh 157 pounds, your BMI would be 27, whether you are male or female.

Your BMI Category

Everyone falls into one of the four BMI categories, as shown in the box below.

If your BMI is less than 18.5, you may weigh too little for optimum health. If your BMI is 18.5 to 24.9, you are in the healthy BMI category. Congratulations—only 35 percent of U.S. adults have a healthy BMI. If you're one of them, your goal is to keep it healthy by not gaining weight. The small changes promoted by the Step Diet can help. If your BMI is between 25 and 29.9, you are in the overweight category. The bad news here is that your risk of developing a chronic disease such as type 2 diabetes is increased. The good news is that you are not yet in the obese category, where health risks are much higher. Think of yourself as approaching the danger zone. Your weight is probably creeping up; if you continue to gain a little more each year, you will soon be in the obese category.

ADULT CLASSIFICATIONS OF OVERWEIGHT

CLASSIFICATION	BMI (KG/M^2)
Underweight	<18.5
Healthy range	18.5–24.9
Overweight	25–29.9
Obese	≥30

Modest weight loss can reduce your risk of developing a chronic disease and make you feel better about yourself.

If your BMI is 30 or above, you are in the obese category. Your weight is clearly too high, and it puts you at much increased risk of developing a chronic disease. You do not need to get your BMI all the

WHAT ABOUT KIDS?

Growth charts are available for children under the age of eighteen at www.cdc.gov (search for clinical growth charts). Your pediatrician can plot your child's BMI on these charts in a way that determines whether he or she is gaining too much weight. Make sure to ask your pediatrician to do this.

way down to the healthy category in order to improve your health. Even modest weight loss can reduce your risk of developing type 2 diabetes, heart disease, and cancer.

It is important to know which BMI category you are in; this helps you understand the relative risk that your weight presents for your health. You are likely reading this book because you are concerned about your BMI. Either you want to lose weight (lower your BMI), or you want to avoid gaining weight (keep your BMI from increasing). If you are an adult, the only way to change your BMI is to change your weight, and the only way to change your weight permanently is to change your lifestyle.

The Cost to Your Health

Clearly, being overweight is not just a cosmetic problem; it also increases your risks of developing a number of chronic diseases that can lead to premature death—including type 2 diabetes, heart disease, and many forms of cancer. Obesity and type 2 diabetes are very closely related, because excess body fat interferes with your body's ability to produce and use the hormone insulin, which helps process sugars. Similarly, excess body fat (particularly if it is around your middle)

BODY MASS INDEX TABLE

	Healthy						*Overweight*					*Obese*					

BMI	19	20	21	22	23	24	25	26	27	28	29	30	31	32	33	34	35	36
HEIGHT (INCHES)							BODY WEIGHT (POUNDS)											
58	91	96	100	105	110	115	119	124	129	134	138	143	148	153	158	162	167	172
59	94	99	104	109	114	119	124	128	133	138	143	148	153	158	163	168	173	178
60	97	102	107	112	118	123	128	133	138	143	148	153	158	163	168	174	179	184
61	100	106	111	116	122	127	132	137	143	148	153	158	164	169	174	180	185	190
62	104	109	115	120	126	131	136	142	147	153	158	164	169	175	180	186	191	196
63	107	113	118	124	130	135	141	146	152	158	163	169	175	180	186	191	197	203
64	110	116	122	128	134	140	145	151	157	163	169	174	180	186	192	197	204	209
65	114	120	126	132	138	144	150	156	162	168	174	180	186	192	198	204	210	216
66	118	124	130	136	142	148	155	161	167	173	179	186	192	198	204	210	216	223
67	121	127	134	140	146	153	159	166	172	178	185	191	198	204	211	217	223	230
68	125	131	138	144	151	158	164	171	177	184	190	197	203	210	216	223	230	236
69	128	135	142	149	155	162	169	176	182	189	196	203	209	216	223	230	236	243
70	132	139	146	153	160	167	174	181	188	195	202	209	216	222	229	236	243	250
71	136	143	150	157	165	172	179	186	193	200	208	215	222	229	236	243	250	257
72	140	147	154	162	169	177	184	191	199	206	213	221	228	235	242	250	258	265
73	144	151	159	166	174	182	189	197	204	212	219	227	235	242	250	257	265	272
74	148	155	163	171	179	186	194	202	210	218	225	233	241	249	256	264	272	280
75	152	160	168	176	184	192	200	208	216	224	232	240	248	256	264	272	279	287
76	156	164	172	180	189	197	205	213	221	230	238	246	254	263	271	279	287	295

Source: Adapted from *Clinical Guidelines on the Identification, Evaluation, and Treatment of Overweight and Obesity in Adults: The Evidence Report.*

BODY MASS INDEX TABLE

Extremely Obese

37	38	39	40	41	42	43	44	45	46	47	48	49	50	51	52	53	54
								BODY WEIGHT (POUNDS)									
177	181	186	191	196	201	205	210	215	220	224	229	234	239	244	248	253	258
183	188	193	198	203	208	212	217	222	227	232	237	242	247	252	257	262	267
189	194	199	204	209	215	220	225	230	235	240	245	250	255	261	266	271	276
195	201	206	211	217	222	227	232	238	243	248	254	259	264	269	275	280	285
202	207	213	218	224	229	235	240	246	251	256	262	267	273	278	284	289	295
208	214	220	225	231	237	242	248	254	259	265	270	278	282	287	293	299	304
215	221	227	232	238	244	250	256	262	267	273	279	285	291	296	302	308	314
222	228	234	240	246	252	258	264	270	276	282	288	294	300	306	312	318	324
229	235	241	247	253	260	266	272	278	284	291	297	303	309	315	322	328	334
236	242	249	255	261	268	274	280	287	293	299	306	312	319	325	331	338	344
243	249	256	262	269	276	282	289	295	302	308	315	322	328	335	341	348	354
250	257	263	270	277	284	291	297	304	311	318	324	331	338	345	351	358	365
257	264	271	278	285	292	299	306	313	320	327	334	341	348	355	362	369	376
265	272	279	286	293	301	308	315	322	329	338	343	351	358	365	372	379	386
272	279	287	294	302	309	316	324	331	338	346	353	361	368	375	383	390	397
280	288	295	302	310	318	325	333	340	348	355	363	371	378	386	393	401	408
287	295	303	311	319	326	334	342	350	358	365	373	381	389	396	404	412	420
295	303	311	319	327	335	343	351	359	367	375	383	391	399	407	415	423	431
304	312	320	328	336	344	353	361	369	377	385	394	402	410	418	426	435	443

increases the chances that you will develop heart disease and cancer. (Most types of cancer are more prevalent in those who are overweight than in those with a healthy BMI.) Obesity is a public health problem and a major reason why our health care costs are skyrocketing. Many experts argue that being overweight is even a more serious threat to people's health than cigarette smoking.

If you look at the figure below, you can see that as BMI increases, the risk of mortality (dying from any cause) increases. When the mortality ratio is above 1, this means the risk of dying is increased above "normal"; when it is below 1, it means the risk of dying is decreased below "normal." Not every person with a higher BMI will develop a disease, but the risk does increase. For example, if your BMI is 40, you are 2.5 times more likely to die from a chronic disease than someone with a BMI of less than 25.

Put simply, being overweight increases your risk of high blood pressure; high blood cholesterol; high triglycerides; low HDL cholesterol;

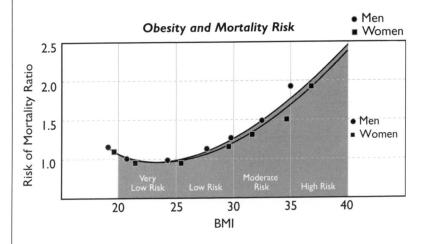

Source: Adapted with permission from Elsevier Inc. Gray DS. *Med Clin North Am.* 1989; 73:1.

developing type 2 diabetes, heart disease, stroke, and some forms of cancer; gallstones; osteoarthritis; sleep apnea; depression; social stigmatization; negative body image; and a reduced quality of life.

Big Around the Waist?

BMI is one measure of your weight problem; waist circumference is another. The bigger your waistline, the more visceral fat you have. Visceral fat is the fat around your internal organs—your liver and kidneys. Fat around your middle is more harmful to your health than fat in other areas of your body. Scientists do not know exactly why this is so, but having

Q. How fast should I lose weight?

A. The National Institutes of Health recommends weight loss of 1 to 2 pounds per week. This means producing a negative energy balance of 500 to 1,000 calories per day. More rapid weight loss has been associated with rapid weight regain.

a lot of fat near your liver, a key organ regulating your metabolism, may have a more negative impact on your health than having fat in other locations. We do know that people with more visceral fat have a higher risk of developing diabetes than those with less visceral fat.

You can find out if you have too much visceral fat simply by measuring your waist circumference. Locate the top of each of your hipbones. Place a measuring tape in a horizontal plane (parallel to the floor) around your middle at the level of the top of your hipbones. Before reading the measuring tape, make sure that it is snug but does not compress your skin. Take your measurement at the end of a normal breath (after you have exhaled).

Don't rely on the waist size of your pants. Many people (particularly men) wear their pants below their waist. You may wear the same size jeans as you did twenty years ago—but you didn't have a big belly flopping over them then!

Managing Chronic Diseases

Frank had always been a little heavy, but he had never worried much about it. Like many people, he did not associate creeping weight gain with increased health risk—even though his father had been overweight much of his life, developed diabetes when he was sixty-two, and died of a heart attack at sixty-six. Frank's weight began to creep up when he was in his thirties—then, at thirty-six, he too was diagnosed with diabetes. This was a major shock to Frank. He was a young man, and now he had a chronic disease that could lead to blindness, limb amputations, and heart disease. Now he had to start taking medication, probably for the rest of his life.

Frank's doctor told him that if he lost 30 pounds he would be better able to manage his diabetes, but neither Frank nor his doctor really expected that to happen. That's because they both knew that losing weight is hard and that most people who do succeed in losing weight eventually gain it back. On the Step Diet, Frank set a reasonable goal of 15 pounds. When he lost the weight and kept it off, he went a long way toward improving his health and his quality of life.

If you are a man, you have too much visceral fat if your waist circumference is more than 40 inches. If you are a woman, you have too much visceral fat if your waist circumference is greater than 35 inches. It does not matter how tall you are.

Obesity experts are trying to get physicians and other health care professionals to routinely measure waist circumference along with BMI.

This combination can be invaluable in determining your health risks. If your BMI is above 30, you are at greatly increased health risk. If your waist circumference is also high, that risk is even higher. If your BMI is less than 30, it is especially useful to know your waist circumference. For example, Joe has a BMI of 28 and a waist circumference of 41 inches. He is at greater risk of developing a chronic disease such as type 2 diabetes than Frank, who has the same BMI but a waist circumference of 36 inches. This is because more of Joe's excess body fat is around his middle.

The good news is that much of the fat that disappears with weight loss comes first from visceral fat. This is why we want you to monitor your waist circumference as you lose weight on the Step Diet.

SUCCESS TIP

Research has shown that people who are regular walkers have a smaller waist circumference than those who do not walk regularly. As you begin walking more, you should see your waist circumference go down—maybe even before you start losing the pounds.

HEALTH BENEFITS OF MODEST WEIGHT LOSS

- Decreased risk of heart disease
- Decreased risk of diabetes
- Decreased risk of some cancers
- Decreased levels of blood glucose (blood sugar) and insulin
- Decreased blood pressure
- Decreased levels of LDL (bad cholesterol) and triglycerides

- Increased HDL (good cholesterol)
- Decrease in severity of sleep apnea
- Reduced symptoms of degenerative joint disease
- Improvement in gynecologic conditions
- Reduced incidence and symptoms of depression

Many people report that they lose inches from their waist even before they lose pounds on the scale. Good job! Losing inches from your waist will bring tremendous benefits.

Overweight Children Get Adult Diseases

"My, how you've grown" is what we usually say about a child's change in height. But nowadays, it could very well be said in recognition of many kids' increased width. Since 1980, the prevalence of overweight has more than doubled in our youth; in some subpopulations of children, the rate of weight gain has been even greater. And despite the wishful thinking of most parents, the vast majority of kids will *not* "grow into" their bodies—80 percent of overweight children become overweight adults.

Perhaps the most frightening aspect of this problem is that obesity among children today is translating into chronic disease—sometimes during youth, often during adulthood. Diagnoses of type 2 diabetes (formerly called adult onset diabetes) among children and adolescents have increased more than tenfold in the past decade alone. The Centers for Disease Control and Prevention has estimated that one out of three children born in the year 2000 will develop diabetes at some point. Imagine a ten-year-old child going on drug therapy or daily insulin injections—and having to continue them for possibly fifty or sixty years. The effects on this child's quality of life will be devastating, and the medical treatment costs staggering. Per person, it costs about $3,000 to $6,000 a year to treat diabetes.

Tragically, other medical woes await many children who are over-weight, including elevated blood pressure, blood choles-terol, and triglyceride levels, which in turn can lead to premature atherosclerosis

> **NOT JUST BABY FAT**
>
> 80 percent of overweight children become overweight adults.

and heart disease. And we're not talking about isolated cases of individual children with rare disorders—this is a fast-spreading health crisis.

Your Weight and Your Quality of Life

B eing overweight can have a devastating impact on your happiness. You may feel discriminated against (and scientific studies show that you are). You are also more likely to be depressed, to have low self-esteem, and to feel that your weight is interfering with your enjoyment of life. While weight loss is not the answer to all your problems, people who have successfully lost weight and kept it off tell us that life is better and that they are happier than they were before the weight loss.

We don't have enough data to know how much weight loss is necessary to improve one's quality of life, but we have found over and over in our twenty-five years of research that people feel better about themselves and report a better quality of life even with a weight loss of 5 to 10 percent.

The Importance of Physical Fitness

You may have read in the newspaper about the "fitness versus fatness" debate in the scientific community. A few scientists have argued that obesity, per se, is not a health risk. Rather, they hold low physical fitness accountable for all the health risks of obesity. Few obesity experts agree with this notion, since we have a great deal of information that links obesity with poor health. The point is, however, that being more physically fit will improve your health whatever your weight and BMI.

This is a very important concept for you to grasp as you set your weight-management goals. If you increase your physical activity and become more physically fit—even if you don't change your weight or your BMI—you will improve your health. You will lower your risk of

FITNESS VERSUS FATNESS

Increasing physical activity, even without weight loss, can greatly improve your health and happiness.

developing a chronic disease, and you will be better able to manage an existing chronic disease. Simply getting more physically active is a great goal by itself.

Losing Weight to Look Better

Wanting to look or feel better is a common reason for people to lose weight. Let's face it, we are all concerned about our appearance, and we all think we look better when we are thinner. Be cautious, however, if you want to lose weight quickly in order to look good for some upcoming event. It is possible to lose weight quickly, but that is not what the Step Diet is about. We would prefer that you take your time and learn the right way to lose weight. You may not look as good as you would like for the upcoming event, but think of all those future events when you will *still* look great.

Success Story 7

Not a Lean Machine, but Living Like One

Bob had a BMI of 36, which he reduced to 33 with the Step Diet. He usually takes more than 11,000 steps per day, and he is feeling good. He would like to lose more weight, but he has reached a zone he is comfortable with. Is Bob still obese? Yes, but he has dramatically improved his health by losing weight and increasing his physical activity.

How Much Weight Loss Is Feasible for You?

The body weight you will be able to maintain permanently will represent a balance among three factors: your genes, your behavior, and the environment in which you live. We want you to consider each of these factors before developing your personal weight goal. Additionally, your weight-management goal will likely be a compromise between the weight you would ideally like to be and the weight that is feasible for you to maintain.

Genetics: Play the Cards You Are Dealt

You might dream of looking like one of the models on the cover of a fashion magazine. Is this likely to happen? Probably not, because we have to work with the genes that we inherited, and most of us have not inherited fashion model genes. Does this mean you are doomed to be overweight? Absolutely not!

On the other hand, don't fall into the trap of blaming your weight problem solely on your genes. Scientists have identified many genes that can affect weight, and there may be many more we do not know about. Your weight could easily be influenced by hundreds of genes, each playing a small role. But only in rare cases does that complex combination of genes doom anyone to be overweight.

Think of your genes as determining the range of body

> **FACT**
>
> Genes do influence body weight but rarely doom anyone to being overweight.

weight that is possible for you. Where you are within that genetically possible range depends on the environment in which you live and the lifestyle you choose within that environment. You can be at the high end of your genetic range of weight or at the low end—and the Step Diet can help you get to the low end.

Your genetic range may be quite wide—for a big man it could be as great as 300 pounds. Or it could be much narrower, encompassing, say, only 50 pounds. The point is that, within your genetic range, you can—and should—achieve a healthy body weight.

Of course, there is currently no way for you to know exactly what weight range is genetically possible for you. But you can get a general sense of it by considering your lowest and highest adult weights (not including pregnancy). Your genetic weight range is certainly at least this broad. Knowing this can help you understand that setting a goal significantly below your lowest adult body weight may not be reasonable.

No matter what your genetic pattern, though, changing your body weight is still about energy balance. If you match energy in and energy out, you will keep a constant body weight. If you eat less energy than you burn, you will lose weight. Here is where your genes can come into play: They can influence how much or how quickly you lose weight when you are in negative energy balance.

Genes may also help explain why some people seem to gain or lose weight more easily than others. Everyone loses weight when they are in a state of negative energy balance, but some people may lose a little more than others.

GENETICS AT WORK

Even though they weighed about the same and had the same BMI, Barbara lost 30 pounds on the Step Diet and Anna lost only 18. Both were happy with their weight loss, but Anna felt that it was unfair that she switched to the same lifestyle as Barbara, yet lost less weight. But it's important for Anna to know what is a realistic weight for her, not for Barbara.

One final point about genes and body weight: Genes have played the lesser part in the growing tendency toward overweight over the past few decades. Our genes have not changed over the last thirty years. Our lifestyle has.

Behavior: Change It, Change Your Weight

Through your own behavior—by making better choices about what and how much you eat and about your physical activity patterns—you can permanently change your weight. Commonly, those changes are temporary, but with the Step Diet, you can make small behavior changes that can be maintained over time, thus leading to permanent changes in weight.

Your current weight is a result of behavioral choices you have made in the past about your eating and physical activity patterns. If you are like most people, you have found it difficult to push back against the environment to keep from passively overeating and from being sedentary. You are probably gaining a little weight each year.

Your genes and your behavior interact to influence your weight. This is a simple relationship but one that few people understand. You come to the table (so to speak) with the genes you inherited. If you are lucky, you have inherited genes that make it easy for you to keep a healthy body weight. Sara is pretty lucky. Even without paying attention to her behavior, she gained only a small amount of weight between the ages of twenty and forty. Betty, on the other hand, is very susceptible to gaining weight and put on 75 pounds during the same period. If both Sara and Betty engage in regular physical activity and eat smart, both will benefit. Sara will be able to keep from gaining any weight, while Betty will still gain weight—but 50 fewer pounds!

Environment: A Big Player

Your eating and physical activity behaviors do not occur in a vacuum. The environment in which you live influences what you choose to eat and how

Q. I am the only person in my family who has a weight problem. If my family members all came from the same gene pool, how come I am the only one who has a hard time controlling my weight?

A. Genes don't tell the whole story; we have to look at the environment we live in as well as the role food may play for us in dealing with emotions and stress. Your weight struggle is related to how you respond uniquely to your environment. Ultimately, this comes down to how much you eat in relation to how much you move.

much and what kind of physical activity you choose to engage in, making it an important factor in determining how you meet your weight-management goal. Or, put another way, your genes are not changeable, your behavior is totally changeable, and your environment is partially changeable.

Let's consider some ways in which your environment affects your behavior. A big part of the Step Diet is getting you to permanently increase the amount you walk. In order to do this, you must have time to walk and a place to walk. Your environment can make this easy or hard. For example, Joanie works for a company that encourages its employees to go out and walk during morning and afternoon breaks and at lunch, and there is even an incentive program to reward employees who reach specific walking goals. Joanie also lives in a traditional community with sidewalks and neighborhood stores. Making time and finding places to walk are not barriers for her.

Helen, on the other hand, works for an employer who counts the minutes of her breaks and pushes her to spend more time at her computer. When she goes home, it is to a suburban neighborhood with cul-de-sacs and no sidewalks. The grocery store is about a mile away, separated from her house by six lanes of traffic on a highway without crosswalks.

Even if Joanie and Helen have the same motivation to walk more,

Helen will obviously have a harder time reaching the goal. Can Helen change her environment? Maybe, to some extent. She may not have control over where she works, and she may not be able to afford to move to a walkable neighborhood. She might, however, try to make changes to her current work and home environment that would help reinforce her goal of increased walking. She might identify places she can walk before or after work. She might find a neighborhood near her own to which she could drive and then take a walk. She might even try to convince her employer to change his attitude toward walking by showing him that physically active employees cost less in health care.

People's food environments differ, too. For example, Jim travels a lot for work and is always eating out. He's often in a hurry, so he does not always have the opportunity to eat at a place that offers healthy choices. His food intake can vary widely from one day to the next. Fred, on the other hand, rarely travels for work. Healthy eating is an important priority for his wife, who prepares most of their meals. They have a lot of consistency in the types of food they eat during the week. While both Jim and Fred can do well with the Step Diet, eating less may present a greater challenge for Jim because of his food environment. Can Jim change his food environment? Again, the answer is maybe. He may not be able to get a job that does not involve travel. He can, however, look for restaurants that offer healthier choices.

Almost certainly, some things in your environment are changeable. Let's start with your physical activity. Can you change how you travel to work? Can you park your car farther away from your building, or if you use public transit, can you find a way to permanently build in some walking each day (say, by getting off the bus or train a few stops earlier)? Can you find ways to replace short trips by car (less than one mile) with walking? Can you start a walking group at work? If these changes become part of your routine, you have changed your environment.

You might also consider how to change your food environment. Here is where it might be helpful to turn back to the food records you kept before starting the Step Diet. Take a look to see how you might modify your food environment. Pay close attention to the times you engaged in passive overeating. Were these at particular times or in particular places? Did you overeat primarily at home or when eating out? You might be able to avoid passive overeating by making simple changes in your food environment. Do you routinely eat at restaurants that serve large portions? Can you find alternative restaurants where portion sizes are more reasonable? You might also examine the types of snack foods you keep around the house and at work. Are you keeping foods that discourage passive overeating?

Setting Your Initial Weight-Loss Goal

We have given you a lot to think about. You now know that your genes can affect how much weight you will lose and how much you can keep off. Your genes can even affect how difficult it is for you to lose weight. It isn't fair, but that's life. You also know that whatever your genetic pattern, you can change your weight by changing your behavior. The more you change your behavior, the more weight you can keep off permanently. You know that your environment affects your behavior and your weight. Your environment may or may not be a barrier to making small lifestyle changes. Finally, you know that increasing your physical activity level will improve your health, no matter what your weight and BMI are, now or in the future.

Now it is time for you to think seriously about your weight-loss goal. If you are already in the healthy weight category, your current weight is your goal. (You still might want to lose a few pounds, which is fine, but be careful not to overdo it.) If you are in the overweight or obese category, it will be useful for you to write down your weight-loss goals. You should make these goals known to those who will help and support you as you begin losing weight.

> **STEP COUNTERS ARE INFECTIOUS**
>
> Tell those around you how much fun step counters are and get them going on the Step Diet. You can convert the neighborhood, your book club, or your church.

We suggest that your initial weight loss goal be between 5 and 15 percent of your current weight. Losing 5 percent of your initial weight and keeping it off is a very achievable goal for most people. Losing 15 percent of your initial weight and keeping it off is a much harder goal. You should decide where in this range your initial goal should be.

The chart below shows how Jeannie, who is 5 feet 6, would calculate what 5 to 15 percent of her current weight would be and how this much weight loss would affect her BMI (as shown on pages 48–49).

Now you will want to do the same computation for yourself, using the chart on page 64. Begin by entering your current weight in the blank on the left. Then calculate how much weight you would have to lose to achieve a 5 percent, 10 percent, or 15 percent weight loss. Enter these

JEANNIE'S POSSIBLE WEIGHT-LOSS GOALS

	PERCENTAGE OF WEIGHT TO LOSE			
CURRENT WEIGHT	5%	10%	15%	20%
192 lbs BMI = 31	9.6 lbs BMI = 29	19.2 lbs BMI = 28	28.8 lbs BMI = 26	38.4 lbs BMI = 25

(Explanation: 5 percent of 192 lbs = 192 × .05 = 9.6 lbs and so on)

YOUR PERSONAL WEIGHT-LOSS GOALS

PERCENTAGE OF WEIGHT TO LOSE

CURRENT WEIGHT/ BMI	5%	10%	15%	20%
____ lbs BMI = ___	____ lbs BMI = ___	____ lbs BMI = ___	____ lbs BMI = ___	____ lbs BMI = ___

Your initial weight-loss goal: _____ pounds
Your initial BMI target: _____

---

numbers in the appropriate blanks in the chart. On the Step Diet you will lose up to 2 pounds per week over the twelve weeks (for a maximum of 24 pounds) of the program. This is the medically recommended healthy rate of weight loss, and this is the rate that leads to greater long-term success. You can lose additional weight by repeating Stages 3–6 of the Step Diet, but first you must determine whether you can maintain your initial weight loss. Choose an initial goal that is from 5 to 15 percent of your current body weight and that is no greater than 24 pounds. It is normal to revise your goals as you progress with weight loss. If you change your weight loss goal, come back to these tables to recalculate your timeline for achieving your goal and to determine the impact on your BMI.

Are You Willing to Do What It Takes?

Now you have considered why you want to lose weight and how much weight loss is feasible for you. The next big question is whether you are prepared to do what it takes to achieve your goals. Losing weight and keeping it off is not easy. You cannot continue to live your current lifestyle and expect your weight to change. The Step Diet shows you how to lose weight and keep it off by making small changes in how much you eat and how much you move. These are achievable changes for most people, but they are still changes. We will show you what to do, but you must be ready to do what it takes.

How Will You Measure Success?

Another reason to be specific about your weight-loss goals is so you can have another measure of success, not just pounds lost. For example, if you want to lose weight to improve your health, you can monitor your success by having your lipids, blood pressure, and other risk factors measured by your physician. You will likely get big improvements in your health with modest weight loss. Similarly, consider measuring success by how much better you feel and how much better you are able to move around. It is fine to have weight loss as one measure of success, but consider having others as well.

Twelve Weeks

Most diets let you try to lose weight for as long as you want. Usually, however, most of your weight loss happens early in your program, then slows or stops after a while. This is both because your body's metabolism is slowing down and because you get tired of changing and restricting the foods

Q. How long will it take to reach my weight-loss goal?

A. You can expect to lose about 1 to 2 pounds per week on the Step Diet. This is the rate of weight loss that gives you the best chance of keeping your weight off permanently. Now that you have a weight-loss target, you can calculate how long it will take you to reach your goal. If your weight-loss goal is greater than 24 pounds, you may need to complete additional twelve-week cycles of weight loss on the Step Diet.

you eat. Your weight loss will be much more effective if you diet for a defined period of time. Twelve weeks is long enough for you to lose enough weight to make a difference in your health and your quality of life, but not so long that you get tired of the small changes.

After the twelve-week weight-loss period, we will show you how to keep this weight off with an individualized weight maintenance plan. Once you feel confident that you can keep the weight off, you can go through another twelve-week weight-loss cycle.

To visualize your possible weight loss, you can make a graph like the one we've constructed for Wendy, who weighs 250 pounds and wants to lose 50 pounds (20 percent of her body weight). She won't reach her goal weight during her first weight-loss cycle. The graph illustrates Wendy's weight loss at 1 pound per week and at 2 pounds per week. She can plot her weight each week and, as long as it falls between the dotted lines, she is on target.

WENDY'S WEIGHT LOSS OVER 12 WEEKS

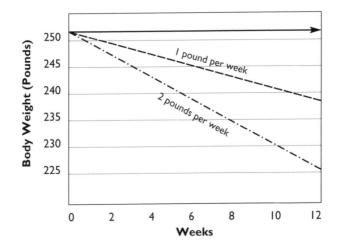

Now make your own chart, using the grid below.

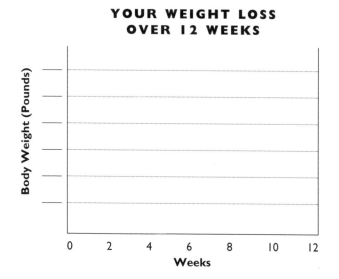

YOUR WEIGHT LOSS
OVER 12 WEEKS

1. Write your current weight (in pounds) in the top blank. (For Wendy, this was 250 pounds.) Subtract 5 pounds and put this number in the blank second from the top. (For Wendy, this was 245 pounds.) Subtract 5 pounds in each lower blank.

2. Subtract 24 pounds from your current weight. (For Wendy, this was 226 pounds.) This is what you would weigh if you lost 2 pounds each week during the twelve-week weight-loss cycle. Put a dot at this level, above the twelve-week value. Draw a line from this value to your starting weight, ending above the 0 time point.

3. Subtract 12 pounds from your current weight. (For Wendy, this was 238 pounds.) This is what you would weigh if you lost 1 pound each week during the twelve-week weight-loss cycle. Put a dot at this level, and above the twelve-week value. Draw a line from this value to your starting weight, ending above the 0 time point.

4. Each week, plot your weight above the appropriate time value.

5. You are on target if your weight stays between the two lines.

Setting Your Step Goal

We told you earlier that we would show you how to keep losing weight after your initial weight loss. You do this by determining your current total energy expenditure in steps per day so that you can then develop a plan for increasing your physical activity to make up for your drop in metabolism. Your first task is to determine how many steps it takes you right now to burn 1 calorie. (The larger your body, the fewer steps it takes to burn 1 calorie.) Look at the Steps per Calorie tables on pages 72–75. Simply find your height along the top (of either the women's or men's table). Move down in that column until you reach the row that corresponds to your weight along the side. This value is the number of steps it takes you to burn one calorie. Write that number here:

I burn 1 calorie in _____ steps.

Step Diet Terminology

Before we start, you need to learn the new language of energy balance. The important terms are BodySteps, LifeSteps, and MegaSteps. These terms will help you to monitor your energy balance and take control of your own body weight. Remember that you will be more successful thinking of energy balance in terms of steps rather than in terms of calories, because unlike calories, you can measure steps accurately.

Your total energy expenditure is the sum of your body's metabolism and your physical activity. When we convert the energy you burn through your body's resting metabolism into steps, we call them BodySteps —the steps your body *does* for you. When you add BodySteps to the steps you measure on your step counter (and adding in the step value of any physical activity not measured by your step counter), you get what we call LifeSteps—the steps you accumulated during an active lifestyle. When we add BodySteps to LifeSteps (the total energy your body burns), the number can get fairly large—hence, the necessity for MegaSteps. A MegaStep is simply 1,000 steps; 37,000 steps equals 37 MegaSteps.

Calculating Your Energy Expenditure in Steps

1. Use the BodyStep tables in Appendix B (pages 180–235) to find your BodySteps. Find the table for your gender and age, then find your height along the top and your weight along the side. The value that corresponds to your height and weight will be the number of steps associated with your metabolism based on your body size. This is your personal BodySteps value.

I get ____ BodySteps.

2. Record the average number of steps you get each day from your step counter. This should include the 2,000 increase you made earlier to stop weight gain.

I get ____ steps per day from my step counter.

3. Record the average number of steps you get each day from activities not measured by your step counter, such as swimming or biking. You can get the step equivalents for these activities on pages 98–99. Remember, this should be the average you get each day.

I get ____ steps per day from activities such as swimming or cycling that are not measured by my step counter.

4. Add the numbers for 2 and 3 above to get your total daily LifeSteps.

I get ____ LifeSteps per day.

5. Add your BodySteps and your LifeSteps to get your total steps.

I get ____ total steps per day.

6. Divide your total for number 5 by 1,000 (you can just move the decimal three places to the left) to get the number of daily MegaSteps you get.

I get ____ MegaSteps per day.

Your MegaSteps per day total is a good estimate of your total energy expenditure. Your goal is to keep this number constant as you lose weight. To do this, you will increase your LifeSteps to compensate for the expected drop in your BodySteps, because of the drop in your metabolism when you lose weight. We will show you how to do this in the next chapter.

Your Physical Activity Percentage

We want you to make one additional calculation that will be useful in helping you keep your weight off. Simply divide your LifeSteps (from number 4) by your total daily steps (number 5) and multiply this number by 100. This will tell you the proportion of your total energy expenditure that comes from physical activity (LifeSteps.)

I get ____ percent of my energy expenditure from physical activity.

Let's use Lynn as an example. She is forty-four years old. She weighs 180 pounds and is 5 feet, 5 inches tall. Her average number of LifeSteps per day is 5,600.

1. Lynn's energy expenditure at rest is 30,301 BodySteps/day (from p. 193 in the tables in Appendix B).

2. Lynn does 5,600 LifeSteps.

3. Lynn gets no physical activity that is not measured by her step counter.

4. Lynn's total energy expenditure is 30,301 BodySteps + 5,600 LifeSteps = 35,901 total daily steps.

5. Lynn gets 36 MegaSteps (35,901 ÷ 1,000).

6. The percentage of total energy expenditure that comes from physical activity is 5,600 divided by 35,901 × 100 or 15.6 percent. If we round this up, Lynn burns 16 percent of her total daily energy during physical activity and 84 percent of her daily energy at rest.

Most overweight people burn substantially less than 25 percent of their total energy expenditure while engaging in physical activity. Scientific studies have shown that people who are this sedentary have a very high risk of gaining weight. Your chances of successfully maintaining a weight loss are very small if you burn less than 25 percent of your total energy expenditure through physical activity. This is why we put so much focus on getting you to move more. By the end of the Step Diet, you will be burning more than 25 percent of your energy expenditure during physical activity. This will greatly increase your chances of successful, long-term weight management.

STEPS PER CALORIE
Women

Weight	Height						
	4'10"	4'11"	5'0"	5'1"	5'2"	5'3"	5'4"
100	40	39	38	38	37	37	36
105	38	37	37	36	35	35	34
110	36	35	35	34	34	33	33
115	34	34	33	33	32	32	31
120	33	32	32	31	31	30	30
125	32	31	31	30	30	29	29
130	31	30	29	29	29	28	28
135	29	29	28	28	27	27	27
140	28	28	27	27	26	26	26
145	27	27	26	26	26	25	25
150	26	26	26	25	25	24	24
155	26	25	25	24	24	24	23
160	25	24	24	24	23	23	22
165	24	24	23	23	22	22	22
170	23	23	23	22	22	21	21
175	23	22	22	22	21	21	21
180	22	22	21	21	21	20	20
185	21	21	21	20	20	20	19
190	21	21	20	20	20	19	19
195	20	20	20	19	19	19	18
200	20	19	19	19	19	18	18
205	19	19	19	18	18	18	18
210	19	19	18	18	18	17	17
215	18	18	18	18	17	17	17
220	18	18	17	17	17	17	16
225	18	17	17	17	16	16	16
230	17	17	17	16	16	16	16
235	17	17	16	16	16	16	15
240	17	16	16	16	15	15	15
245	16	16	16	15	15	15	15
250	16	16	15	15	15	15	14
255	16	15	15	15	15	14	14
260	15	15	15	15	14	14	14
265	15	15	14	14	14	14	14
270	15	14	14	14	14	14	13
275	14	14	14	14	13	13	13
280	14	14	14	13	13	13	13
285	14	14	13	13	13	13	13
290	14	13	13	13	13	13	12
295	13	13	13	13	13	12	12
300	13	13	13	13	12	12	12

STEPS PER CALORIE
Women

5'5"	5'6"	5'7"	5'8"	5'9"	5'10"	5'11"	6'0"
35	35	34	34	33	33	32	32
34	33	33	32	32	31	31	30
32	32	31	31	30	30	29	29
31	30	30	29	29	29	28	28
29	29	29	28	28	27	27	27
28	28	27	27	27	26	26	26
27	27	26	26	26	25	25	25
26	26	25	25	25	24	24	24
25	25	25	24	24	23	23	23
24	24	24	23	23	23	22	22
24	23	23	23	22	22	22	21
23	22	22	22	22	21	21	21
22	22	21	21	21	21	20	20
21	21	21	20	20	20	20	19
21	20	20	20	20	19	19	19
20	20	20	19	19	19	19	18
20	19	19	19	19	18	18	18
19	19	19	18	18	18	18	17
19	18	18	18	18	17	17	17
18	18	18	17	17	17	17	16
18	17	17	17	17	16	16	16
17	17	17	16	16	16	16	16
17	17	16	16	16	16	15	15
16	16	16	16	16	15	15	15
16	16	16	15	15	15	15	15
16	15	15	15	15	15	14	14
15	15	15	15	14	14	14	14
15	15	15	14	14	14	14	14
15	15	14	14	14	14	13	13
14	14	14	14	14	13	13	13
14	14	14	14	13	13	13	13
14	14	13	13	13	13	13	13
14	13	13	13	13	13	12	12
13	13	13	13	13	12	12	12
13	13	13	13	12	12	12	12
13	13	12	12	12	12	12	12
13	12	12	12	12	12	12	11
12	12	12	12	12	12	11	11
12	12	12	12	11	11	11	11
12	12	12	11	11	11	11	11
12	12	11	11	11	11	11	11

STEPS PER CALORIE
Men

Weight	Height 5'2"	5'3"	5'4"	5'5"	5'6"	5'7"	5'8"
130	28	28	28	27	27	26	26
135	27	27	26	26	26	25	25
140	26	26	26	25	25	24	24
145	25	25	25	24	24	24	23
150	25	24	24	23	23	23	22
155	24	23	23	23	22	22	22
160	23	23	22	22	22	21	21
165	22	22	22	21	21	21	20
170	22	21	21	21	20	20	20
175	21	21	20	20	20	20	19
180	21	20	20	20	19	19	19
185	20	20	19	19	19	18	18
190	19	19	19	19	18	18	18
195	19	19	18	18	18	18	17
200	18	18	18	18	17	17	17
205	18	18	17	17	17	17	16
210	18	17	17	17	17	16	16
215	17	17	17	16	16	16	16
220	17	17	16	16	16	16	15
225	16	16	16	16	15	15	15
230	16	16	16	15	15	15	15
235	16	15	15	15	15	15	14
240	15	15	15	15	14	14	14
245	15	15	15	14	14	14	14
250	15	15	14	14	14	14	13
255	14	14	14	14	14	13	13
260	14	14	14	14	13	13	13
265	14	14	13	13	13	13	13
270	14	13	13	13	13	13	12
275	13	13	13	13	13	12	12
280	13	13	13	13	12	12	12
285	13	13	13	12	12	12	12
290	13	13	12	12	12	12	12
295	13	12	12	12	12	12	11
300	12	12	12	12	12	11	11
305	12	12	12	12	11	11	11
310	12	12	12	11	11	11	11

STEPS PER CALORIE
Men

5'9"	5'10"	5'11"	6'0"	6'1"	6'2"	6'3"	6'4"	6'5"
26	25	25	24	24	24	23	23	23
25	24	24	24	23	23	23	22	22
24	23	23	23	22	22	22	22	21
23	23	22	22	22	21	21	21	21
22	22	21	21	21	21	20	20	20
21	21	21	21	20	20	20	19	19
21	20	20	20	20	19	19	19	19
20	20	20	19	19	19	18	18	18
20	19	19	19	18	18	18	18	17
19	19	18	18	18	18	17	17	17
18	18	18	18	17	17	17	17	17
18	18	17	17	17	17	16	16	16
17	17	17	17	17	16	16	16	16
17	17	17	16	16	16	16	15	15
17	16	16	16	16	15	15	15	15
16	16	16	16	15	15	15	15	15
16	16	15	15	15	15	15	14	14
15	15	15	15	15	14	14	14	14
15	15	15	14	14	14	14	14	14
15	15	14	14	14	14	14	13	13
14	14	14	14	14	13	13	13	13
14	14	14	14	13	13	13	13	13
14	14	13	13	13	13	13	13	12
14	13	13	13	13	13	12	12	12
13	13	13	13	13	12	12	12	12
13	13	13	12	12	12	12	12	12
13	13	12	12	12	12	12	12	11
13	12	12	12	12	12	12	11	11
12	12	12	12	12	11	11	11	11
12	12	12	12	11	11	11	11	11
12	12	12	11	11	11	11	11	11
12	11	11	11	11	11	11	11	10
11	11	11	11	11	11	11	10	10
11	11	11	11	11	10	10	10	10
11	11	11	11	10	10	10	10	10
11	11	11	10	10	10	10	10	10
11	11	10	10	10	10	10	10	10

WHY BURNING MORE THAN 25 PERCENT OF YOUR TOTAL ENERGY EXPENDITURE IN PHYSICAL ACTIVITY HELPS WITH WEIGHT MANAGEMENT

Physical activity is the part of your body's energy expenditure that you have most control over. Remember, the more physical activity you can get in your day, the less you have to restrict your food intake—and restricting food intake is very hard for people. If you are getting less than 25 percent of your total energy expenditure in physical activity, it is going to be difficult for you to keep from gaining weight without substantial food restriction.

Don't just stop at 25 percent! The higher the proportion of your energy expenditure coming from physical activity, the greater your chances of keeping your weight off. If you are having trouble finding enough time to get all of your daily steps in walking, try a more intense physical activity. You can burn more steps in a shorter time.

CHAPTER 5

Start Losing Weight

Stage 4:
Make small changes to lose weight.

Eat 75 percent of what you normally eat and raise your daily step goal by 500 steps each successive week.

Now you are ready to start losing weight. Over the next twelve weeks (less if you have fewer than 24 pounds to lose), you will eat a little less at each meal and gradually increase your walking. It's that simple. Stick with it, and you will lose 1 to 2 pounds each week, for a total weight loss of 12 to 24 pounds in twelve weeks. (Some people will lose a little less, and some will lose a little more.)

We want you to work hard for twelve weeks, then concentrate on maintaining the weight loss you have achieved. Once you feel comfortable maintaining your new lower weight, you may consider going through another twelve-week weight-loss cycle.

Small Changes, Big Results

The Step Diet allows you to ease into a new lifestyle, rather than overhaul your current one, by encouraging small, achievable changes in what you eat and how much you move. You need to make only two small behavioral changes to lose weight:

> **BECOME A CREATURE OF HEALTHIER HABITS**
>
> Research suggests that it takes about twenty-one days to establish simple behavioral routines. Once you have done something daily for that long, you're likely to continue it without thinking much about it anymore.

1. Eat 75 percent of whatever you are eating right now. Eating 25 percent less is a small change that will probably be easy for you. That's because most of us are already eating much more food than we need or want to, because of passive overeating and typical portions that are at least 25 percent too big for what our bodies need.

TWELVE WEEKS FOR BEST RESULTS

When we reviewed dozens of weight-loss research studies, we found that most of the weight loss occurs in the first twelve weeks, which is why you will just get frustrated if you continue to try to lose weight after twelve weeks. (This is kind of like going to school—you study hard for a semester and then you test yourself before going on to the next level.) Work hard for twelve weeks. Then stop dieting and learn to keep off the weight you lost. Then you can do another twelve-week weight loss period when you are ready. It may take a little longer to lose a lot of weight, but what you lose will stay off.

Actually, a 25 percent reduction is really just taking a step back to adequate portions.

Here is where those food records you completed in Chapter 1 come in handy. How many times during those seven days did you engage in overeating—eating everything on your plate simply because it was there rather than because you wanted it? Reviewing your records of when and where you have typically overeaten may give you clues as to where you can easily implement the 75 percent rule without feeling deprived. The good news is that we are accustomed to eating more than we need, and a 25 percent reduction will not result in feelings of food deprivation.

2. Increase your daily LifeSteps goal by 500 steps during each successive week of the twelve-week weight-loss period. You saw how easy it was to increase your steps by 2,000 a day. We want you to continue to gradually increase the number of steps you take each day. You should aim to raise your daily step goal by 500 steps during each successive week of the weight-loss period. This means that during the first week, you aim for 2,500 additional steps per day above your baseline activity level (this includes the 2,000 steps-per-day increase you did to stop weight gain), 3,000 steps per day during the second week, and so on. By the end of the twelve-week weight-loss period, you will have increased your step goal

Q. **What do I do with the other 25 percent of the food? It seems like such a waste to throw it away.**

A. Most of us were raised not to waste food, so think of today's leftovers as tomorrow's snacks or small meals. Make a sandwich from leftover chicken or pork; use a leftover quarter sandwich from lunch as a snack. If you are serving a family of four, the 25 percent taken off three plates will be enough to fill an entire plate. Add leftover hamburger or steak to a casserole. Or maybe the dog deserves a treat!

by 8,000 steps per day. Increasing your steps will help you in two important ways. First, it burns more energy, helping you lose weight faster. Second, and even more important, it will make up for the drop in metabolic rate (BodySteps) that occurs as you lose weight. This is an important benefit of physical activity, and most weight-loss plans do not explain how it works.

Now, let's look at what happens if you follow the Step Diet to lose weight. Your BodySteps go down because you are becoming smaller, but you make up for this by increasing your LifeSteps. By the end of weight loss, your total energy expenditure (or MegaSteps) will not have declined very much. *That means you will not have to dramatically restrict your food intake to keep your weight off, because you have prevented the decline in your total energy expenditure. This is the secret to long-term weight control.*

Use Your Head Before You Fill Your Mouth

You can undermine your weight-loss efforts if you don't think about what you normally eat during the day—what you need as well as what you cut out. Remember, this plan works best if you don't make big changes to your usual eating pattern. Do not try to save calories by skipping meals or snacks. This could lead to a temporary reduction in energy intake, but it can make you feel so hungry by the next meal that you eat anything that is not nailed down! Eating regular meals and snacks (but eating

Q. I feel like I eat so little anyway, I can't imagine cutting out even a small amount of food.

A. Try this method for at least two weeks and see if you may be eating more than you think. As you increase your physical activity, you may find that your appetite control improves and you actually feel less hungry.

only 75 percent) can help you avoid becoming so hungry that you pile larger portions on your plate or indulge in seconds. Do not decide to eat out more or less frequently during this twelve-week period. Just do what you normally would do. Also, don't make the mistake of assuming that if eating 75 percent is good, eating 50 percent is better—it isn't.

When eating cereal, pour your usual portion in a bowl and then measure it. If you typically eat 2 cups of cereal, put only 1¹/₂ cups into your bowl.

If you maintain your usual eating patterns, the Step Diet plan is simple. Just don't eat 25 percent of your food. No special food, no gimmicks—the only tool you need is a knife to cut your food into quarters so that you can leave one of them behind.

Most main-course foods will be easy to divide into fourths. Hamburgers, hot dogs, pizza, and a variety of sandwiches can easily be cut into four equal sections. Just eat three sections. Many other items, such as casseroles, mashed potatoes, and rice, are also easy to divide into quarters. Some things may take a little more effort. Let's say, for example, you are eating a chicken or turkey leg. Simply cut the meat off the bone and put it on your plate. Then it should be relatively easy to cut it into quarters. When in doubt, you can first put the food on your plate and then quarter it.

It's easy to use the 75 percent rule in fast-food restaurants if you are eating burgers and other sandwiches. For french fries, just estimate what 25 percent would be and don't eat that amount. Shortcuts can also help. If you have always ordered the larger french fries or the bigger burger, start ordering the next smaller size. You have easily saved 25 percent with this simple strategy.

Now, this does not give you license to increase the number of meals you eat at fast-food restaurants. Keep in mind that you are much more likely to get more total energy intake at a restaurant than at home. But

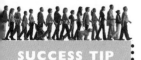

SUCCESS TIP

If you have young children at home, the 25 percent you're not eating makes a great child-sized meal. You'll save money *and* calories!

you can easily use the 75 percent plan in dine-in restaurants. Simply take the 25 percent you leave on your plate home in a doggie bag.

What about special occasions, say, when you are at a party or a buffet? The rule for the Step Diet in these situations is to serve yourself a helping no larger than your fist—then eat 75 percent of this.

Don't forget to downsize your beverages, too. People often underestimate the energy intake they get from what they drink. You must use the 75 percent rule with any beverages that have calories. That excludes only water, diet drinks, and black coffee. If you are pouring your own beverage, just fill the cup or glass three-fourths full. If you are drinking from a can, pour it into a glass and leave one-fourth out. In restaurants, you can take shortcuts, such as ordering a small beverage when you would usually order a large one.

FOOD ITEM	WHOLE PORTION (CALORIES)	75 PERCENT PORTION (CALORIES)
McDonald's Ham, Egg & Cheese Bagel with Hash Browns	680	510
Denny's All-American Slam	710	533
Einstein Bros Santa Fe bagel with eggs	650	488
IHOP Buttermilk Pancakes, full stack with butter and syrup	670	503
Jamba Juice Chocolate Moo'd	690	518

When it comes to snacks, you can use strategies similar to those you used with meals. If there is a smaller portion available, choose it. Buy the small-size popcorn at the movies. If you are popping popcorn at home, leave one-fourth in the bag. If you snack on candy bars, buy the smaller size or just throw away one-fourth. You will find that in most cases it is easy to estimate 75 percent of your snacks.

BEWARE OF CALORIES IN BEVERAGES

Research suggests that our bodies regulate calories in beverages differently than calories in solid foods. You may not feel as full after consuming liquid calories as after consuming solid calories, so it's particularly important that you use the 75 percent rule for your beverages. In fact, you might look for even more ways to avoid beverages that contain calories.

Snacks have received a bad rap over the years, mainly because of what people generally eat for snacks, like potato chips, candy bars, and nuts. You don't have to give these up on the Step Diet, just eat 75 percent of them. You might decide that you occasionally want to substitute a healthier alternative for a snack, like pretzels, fruit, low-fat crackers, string cheese, or a low-calorie energy bar. If you are currently not snacking, don't start unless you find yourself excessively hungry between meals; then try adding one snack each day to see if this helps.

Here are some healthy snack ideas. Just remember to practice the 75 percent portion control rule, because even though these are healthy choices, too much energy intake still leads to weight gain.

- String cheese
- Baked tortilla chips
- Frozen grapes
- Sliced fruit

- Angel food cake
- Frozen fruit juice bars
- Popcorn (light varieties)
- Deli turkey or ham slices
- Gingersnaps
- Energy bar (200 calories or fewer)
- Cottage cheese and mixed fruit
- Fat-free pudding

Free Foods

This is the section that everyone loves—where we list the foods that you can eat any time in any amount. There are no rules for portion control with these choices, because free foods fill you up but don't contain many calories, so that it's nearly impossible to gain weight by overeating them. The best part is that most of them are excellent sources of vitamins, minerals, and fiber.

All vegetables except corn, peas, and dried beans:

- Alfalfa sprouts
- Artichokes
- Asparagus
- Bamboo shoots
- Beets
- Bell peppers
- Bok choy

- Broccoli
- Brussels sprouts
- Cabbage
- Carrots
- Cauliflower
- Celery
- Cucumber

Q. What if I am hungry? I am usually starving when I sit down for a meal.

A. You may be surprised that you won't feel deprived by eating only 75 percent of your food. You might still feel a little hungry when you first stop eating, but a few minutes later (when satiety signals kick in) you may be completely satisfied. The idea behind this type of meal plan is *not* to be excessively hungry. Most people will not stick with a diet if they are hungry. If you find that you are still hungry after cutting out 25 percent of each meal, try adding more "free" foods to your daily intake.

- Eggplant
- Jicama
- Kale
- Lettuce (all types)
- Mushrooms
- Onions
- Parsley

- Radishes
- Spinach
- Squash
- Tomatoes
- Water chestnuts
- Zucchini

The following beverages and desserts are also free foods:

- Black coffee
- Sugar-free Jell-O
- Calorie-free soft drinks
- Starburst Juice Bars
- Club soda

- Kool-Aid Pops
- Crystal Light
- Jell-O Pop Bars
- Unsweetened ice tea

A Typical Day in Your Weight-Loss Week

You may be wondering how you can possibly lose weight just by eating a little less at each meal. Let's look at an example of a typical day and calculate the calories saved by using the 75 percent strategy.

At the rate of over 700 calories a day saved, you will lose almost 1 1/2 pounds per week from managing your portions alone, not including the boost you get from increased walking.

> **CAUTION**
>
> Beware of calories "hitching a ride" with your free foods. If you can, avoid dipping your free foods into salad dressings, butter, margarine, peanut butter, dips, or sauces—all of these can add a lot of fat to your healthy snack. And if you do indulge in these toppings, remember that the 75 percent rule will have to apply.

SAVING CALORIES THE 75 PERCENT WAY

Food	Original Portion Size	Calories	75 Percent	Calorie Savings
Breakfast:				
Large bowl of Cheerios	2 cups	220	1 1/2 cups	55
Skim milk	1/2 cup	45	3/8 cup	11
Coffee, black	1 cup	Free	1 cup	Free
Orange juice	Large glass (8 ounces)	110	Small glass (6 ounces)	28
Snack:				
Doughnut	1 regular	210	3/4 of doughnut	53
Lunch:				
Roast beef sandwich with mayo	1 regular-size sandwich	560	3/4 of sandwich	140
Potato chips	1 small bag	150	3/4 of bag	38
Carrot sticks	4	Free	4	Free
Coke	12-ounce can	150	3/4 of can	38
Snack:				
Milky Way bar	1 regular-size bar	270	3/4 of bar	68
Dinner:				
Tossed salad	2 cups	Free	2 cups	Free
Ranch dressing	2 tablespoons	180	1.5 tablespoons	45
Pork chops	2 medium chops	330	1 1/2 chops	82
Mashed potatoes	1 cup	220	3/4 cup	55
Broccoli, steamed	1 cup	Free	1 cup	Free
Red wine	6-ounce glass	125	4.5 ounces	31
Dessert:				
Bowl of ice cream	1 cup	320	3/4 cup	80

Total calories you would have eaten: 2,890
Total calories you did eat: 2,167
Total calories saved: 723

Checking the MegaStep Value of Your Weight-Loss Diet

In Appendix C on pages 236–270, you will see that we have converted the traditional caloric value of a large number of commonly eaten foods into MegaSteps. The tables may look complicated, but they're not. Next to each food you'll find five columns listing its MegaStep value. You can figure out which column you should use by referring to page 68, where you determined how many steps you need to take to burn 1 calorie of food energy. This value is unique to your sex, height, and weight—and the MegaStep value of each food is likewise unique. For example, if you need to walk 21–25 steps to burn 1 calorie, you would look at the third column in the tables in Appendix C to find the MegaStep value of that food for you.

Although these tables were originally designed to help dieters maintain energy balance *after* they had finished losing weight, we've found them useful to dieters *while* they lose weight too. To begin with, you can use MegaSteps as another way of checking that you are eating 75 percent of your former diet. For example, if your total daily step value (BodySteps plus LifeSteps) is 40,000, or 40 MegaSteps, you know that to keep your weight constant you would need to eat 40 MegaSteps worth of food. If you use the 75 percent strategy, you should be eating 75 percent of 40 MegaSteps (0.75 × 40 MegaSteps), or 30 MegaSteps. Just add up the MegaStep value of the foods that you eat throughout the day to see if you're on target.

These tables may also help you decide between food choices. You might see some easy food substitutions you can make to reduce your energy intake. Just remember not to make too *many* substitutions: The goal is not to reduce your energy intake as much as possible. That strategy does not work. The goal is to eat about 75 percent of what you were eating before.

Why It Works

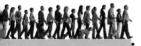

There is no question that most of us could probably improve the quality of our diets, but, for the purpose of managing body weight, by far the most important factor is how much energy we consume in the food we eat. A few years ago, low-fat diets were popular. Now, low-carbohydrate, high-protein diets are popular. Both kinds of diets have been around for centuries, yet we still have an obesity epidemic. Why? Because we are still eating too much food!

Reducing your portion size by 25 percent works. First, it reduces overeating, which is responsible for the weight gain of many people. Second, it is easy to divide food into quarters. Third, it's a specific target for how much less food to eat, not a vague suggestion to "eat less." In addition, cutting your food intake by 25 percent will not trigger a compensatory drop in metabolic rate. And,

THE 75 PERCENT ADVANTAGE

- You can eat all of your favorite foods.

- You won't feel deprived.

- You can still eat out.

- You won't be excessively hungry.

- You can stick with a diet based on small changes.

- You won't experience a drop in metabolic rate.

- You don't have to obsess over what to eat—just eat less of it.

- You can learn to eat less for the rest of your life.

combined with more walking, it will produce a safe and recommended rate of weight loss.

Move More: Increase Your Steps

R emember, your goal is to add 500 extra steps daily during each successive week of the twelve-week weight-loss phase of the Step Diet. In other words, you'll walk 500 more steps per day during the first week, 1,000 more steps per day during the second week, and so on. By the end of the twelve weeks, you will have added 8,000 steps per day (counting the 2,000 you added to stop gaining weight) to your previous total. It sounds like a lot, but it will be easy if you build up your steps gradually. For most of you, this will get your daily step total close to 10,000 or more, which will be sufficient to compensate for the drop in your metabolism that has occurred due to weight loss. Also, it will get you to a point where at least 25 percent of your total energy expenditure comes from physical activity. This is essential for maintaining weight loss.

Every bit of physical activity you perform burns additional energy and will contribute to the state of negative energy balance you are trying to achieve for weight loss. Skipping a big meal and cutting 1,000 calories from your diet is a lot easier than walking the 10 miles it would take to burn 1,000 calories. This is why most weight-loss plans simply concentrate on getting you to eat less. However, if you are going to lose 1 to 2 pounds per week, you must eat 500 to 1,000 fewer calories each day or burn 500 to 1,000 extra calories each day. The best way to do

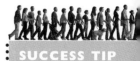

SUCCESS TIP

D on't be an overachiever. If you try to increase your steps by more than 500 a day each week, you might get discouraged. Conversely, don't expect to continue increasing your steps if you've added the 500 just once or twice the previous week. The number of steps has been calibrated so that it will feel like a gradual addition, not a hiker's challenge.

YOUR LIFESTEPS SCHEDULE		
(ADD 500 STEPS PER DAY MORE FOR EACH SUCCESSIVE WEEK.)		
CURRENT STEPS PER DAY _____		
Week 1 _____		Week 7 _____
Week 2 _____		Week 8 _____
Week 3 _____		Week 9 _____
Week 4 _____		Week 10 _____
Week 5 _____		Week 11 _____
Week 6 _____		Week 12 _____

this is by combining eating less and moving more. Remember, this is how more than 90 percent of participants in the National Weight Control Registry lost their weight. The more you restrict your food, the hungrier you are and the more likely you will be to abandon the plan.

You know by now that your resting metabolic rate (your BodySteps) will drop as you lose weight. It will not drop as much initially with small reductions in food intake as with big ones, but it will drop over time as you lose pounds. You can expect your resting metabolic rate to drop by about 8 calories per day for each pound of weight you lose.

We told you earlier in this chapter that this drop in resting metabolic rate often leads people to become frustrated with their weight loss over time. As your resting metabolic rate drops, you will be in progressively less negative energy balance (assuming your degree of food restriction stays the same). This will cause your rate of weight loss to slow down or stop. Then you get frustrated because you are still restricting your food intake but not losing as much weight as before.

Let's take an example. If you lost 50 pounds, we would expect your resting metabolic rate to be 400 calories less per day after your weight

AVOID THE THINGS THAT HAVE TRIPPED YOU UP BEFORE

We developed the Step Diet to help you avoid the common pitfalls that have caused you to fail at losing weight before:

- Inability to manage hunger—since you are eating only a little less, you won't be excessively hungry.

- Drop in metabolic rate—you overcome this by increasing your LifeSteps.

- Diet fatigue—you can lose weight for only twelve weeks, so you don't get sick of dieting.

- Trying to count calories.

- Forgetting about the importance of physical activity.

loss than before. This means that to maintain your new lower body weight by diet alone, you would need to eat 400 fewer calories per day than you were eating before your weight loss—forever. This is why so many people are able to lose weight but not keep it off.

Now, here is where physical activity becomes so important. You would stand a much better chance of keeping your weight off if you could make up for the drop in your metabolism by increasing your physical activity. This is exactly what people in the National Weight Control Registry do. These people report that they spend about sixty minutes each day engaged in various physical activities. While this might seem like more than

FACT

If you lose 30 pounds, your resting metabolic rate will go down by 240 calories per day. For a woman who is 5 feet, 6 inches tall and weighs 180 pounds, this will be a loss of 4,320 BodySteps.

you can manage, remember that much of this comes from walking and can be spread out during the day. We found that people in the National Weight Control Registry take between 11,000 and 13,000 LifeSteps each day. This sounds like a lot, but remember, the average weight loss was more than 65 pounds, and the more weight lost, the more physical activity needed. Your physical activity goal during weight loss is to increase your LifeSteps to make up for the drop in your resting metabolism that occurs as you lose weight. By increasing your LifeStep goal by 500 steps a day each week, you will increase your LifeSteps by 6,000 a day over the twelve-week weight-loss cycle. This increase will completely make up for your drop in resting metabolic rate (BodySteps) and will contribute to your negative energy balance. The bottom line is this: You dramatically increase your chances of being able to keep your weight off if you burn 25 percent of your total daily calories in physical activity. For someone who has a total daily expenditure of 40,000 steps (40 MegaSteps), this means that 10,000 of those steps (10 MegaSteps) come from LifeSteps. Many avid exercisers get 35 percent, 40 percent, or even more energy expenditure from activity. You might notice that these people not only don't have a weight problem, but they seem able to eat anything they want without gaining weight.

Actually, our bodies function better when we are physically active. And part of the reason most people have trouble maintaining energy balance is that their physical activity is so low. When you are very physically inactive, your body is not as capable of balancing energy intake with energy expenditure. When you are physically active, your body helps you maintain energy balance.

To reiterate: Most overweight people burn less than 25 percent of their total energy expenditure during physical activity. Most of their energy expenditure comes from their resting metabolic rate. You have a much

THE LESSONS OF THE MASTERS

Much information in this book was learned from the "Zen masters" of weight management, the folks in the National Weight Control Registry (NWCR). Here are three important statistics that the NWCR has come up with based on reports from thousands of weight controllers. These statistics show why successful weight loss depends on an approach that combines exercise and eating right.

1. Less than 10 percent lost weight with diet alone.

2. Less than 5 percent lost weight with exercise alone.

3. Only 9 percent are keeping their weight off with diet alone.

better chance of maintaining energy balance when at least 25 percent of your total energy expenditure comes from physical activity—which is where you should be at the end of the twelve-week weight-loss cycle. Look back to page 71, where you calculated what percentage of your total energy expenditure comes from LifeSteps. You will recalculate this figure after you complete the twelve-week weight loss cycle.

Let's Walk!

Now that you have a step goal for weight loss and a timetable for reaching that goal, it is time to start walking. We have worked with thousands of people who have used step counters to increase physical activity, and we have learned from them some easy ways to get more steps. (Check out pages 37–42 if you've forgotten the ones we listed earlier.) All you have to do is use your step counter to plan your day the same way you use your watch to keep track of time. For example,

A MILE IS A MILE IS A MILE

You may be surprised to hear that for most people, walking a mile burns the same amount of energy as running a mile—it just takes longer. For any given distance, physics teaches us that the main factor in how much energy you burn is how much you weigh.

let's say that it is 3:00 P.M., you've walked 4,000 steps, and your goal for the day is 10,000 LifeSteps. You must think about the rest of your day and plan how you will fit in the other 6,000 steps.

For example, you might know that you are planning a walk after dinner with your spouse on your favorite 5,000-step route. This means you need only another 1,000 steps. You know you get 300 steps walking to your car. Now you need 700 steps. You know that it is 400 steps down to the cafeteria, and you were planning to walk down for a snack. Walking down and back is 800 steps, so now you have a plan for reaching your step goal.

Steps and Time

People walk at different speeds. In order to find out exactly how many steps you get in a minute of walking, just zero your step counter and go for a ten-minute walk at your usual speed. Then divide the number of steps you get by 10. This information is useful in planning your day. For example, if you walk at 100 steps per minute, and you know you have a 10-minute break in the morning and another in the afternoon, you can plan to get 2,000 steps during these breaks.

It is also extremely useful to know the number of steps you get on some of your favorite walking routes. That way, if you know you need 5,000 steps to reach your goal, and if you know that three times around the block with the dog is about 5,000 steps, you can choose that route for your evening walk.

WHY WALKING?

Shouldn't you run or swim or do something more strenuous for your physical activity? You don't have to with the Step Diet. Here are some reasons why walking is an excellent way to get the physical activity you need to lose weight:

- *Nearly everyone can walk—* even people who have other physical limitations are usually ambulatory.

- *We're all used to walking—it's* by far the biggest contributor to how much energy is expended over and above the resting metabolic rate.

- *Walking requires no special equipment or facilities—*all you need is comfortable clothing and a reliable pair of shoes or sneakers.

- *Walking can be done in a multitude of settings—*you can do it on a street, in the woods, up and down stairs, in a shopping mall . . . virtually anywhere! And it's free.

- *With your step counter, it's easy to measure how much you're walking—*you can figure out how much energy you're burning, which is essential information to manage your energy balance.

List your five favorite walking routes and the number of steps for each.

_____

_____

_____

_____

_____

The U.S. Surgeon General has recommended that every American accumulate at least thirty minutes per day of moderate physical activity (like walking) on most days of the week to stay in peak health. The problem is that it is not easy to know when you have done this. It would be hard to go about your daily activities with a stopwatch, clocking those incidental bursts of walking—climbing a flight of stairs, walking to the drinking fountain, vacuuming the living room—to accumulate your thirty minutes a day. And many people do not have thirty minutes they can set aside to get all of their activity done at once. As a result, lots of people don't even attempt to do more walking. With your step counter, you get credit for every step you take, whether you are just strolling around the house or purposefully power-walking. Every step is a step in the right direction.

Activities Other Than Walking

Your step counter will give you credit for most types of physical activity that involve leg motion, including walking, running, and playing tennis, soccer, and basketball. True, a running step is different from a walking step, but only slightly (most people have a longer stride length when they run than when they walk, resulting in fewer steps per mile), so we treat them the same. However, the steps you take when running or playing tennis can increase your weight loss, because you burn slightly more energy per step in these activities due to your longer stride length.

Because it's impossible for your step counter to measure your energy expenditure for activities such as swimming, weight lifting, and bicycling, we have provided you with a conversion table in case you prefer these activities and do them on a regular basis; see pages 98–99.

Track Your Progress

It is important that you keep track of your progress during the twelve-week weight-loss cycle. Use the chart on page 100 to track the following:

- Body weight
- Waist circumference
- Daily LifeSteps
- Adherence to the 75 percent rule

Many people find it useful to keep track of their progress continually throughout the twelve-week period, while others prefer to do this periodically. Whichever you choose, make sure that you track it with some regularity. Make sure to write down the number of LifeSteps you have accumulated at the end of each day, and check the meals and snacks where you used the 75 percent strategy. You only need to record your weight and waist circumference weekly. Try to do this on the same day at about the same time each week. Because it is important to be aware of what you are eating, we recommend that you complete three days of food records every month during weight loss. Keeping a food record is associated with successful weight management.

If you follow the two simple rules of the Step Diet, you should be shedding pounds and inches. Be proud of yourself! When you have reached a reasonable weight-loss goal, get ready for the next stage: determining your personal energy balance point.

Applying Step Diet Principles to Children and Adolescents

Can the Step Diet work for kids, too? Most definitely, with only a few slight modifications to accommodate actively growing bodies. Of course, we recommend that you consult your pediatrician or family doctor before beginning any diet plan, to make sure that it makes sense for your child.

The key principles of the Step Diet—managing portions to avoid overeating and walking a little more—can work very well for kids. And

STEP EQUIVALENTS OF ACTIVITIES NOT COUNTED BY STEP COUNTERS

WOMEN

ACTIVITY	STEPS PER MINUTE OF ACTIVITY
Canoeing	60
Chopping wood	126
Cycling	150
Horseshoes	52
In-line skating	200
Judo and karate	236
Rowing	150
Skating	150
Skiing:	
Moderate to steep	150
Downhill racing	306
Cross-country	225
Snowshoeing	156
Swimming:	
Pleasure	96
Freestyle—25–50 yards per minute	150
Butterfly—50 yards per minute	256
Backstroke—25–50 yards per minute	150
Breaststroke—25–50 yards per minute	150
Sidestroke—40 yards per minute	196
Volleyball	90
Waterskiing	136
Weight lifting	100
Yoga	50

STEP EQUIVALENTS OF ACTIVITIES NOT COUNTED BY STEP COUNTERS

MEN

ACTIVITY	STEPS PER MINUTE OF ACTIVITY
Canoeing	72
Chopping wood	151
Cycling	180
Horseshoes	62
In-line skating	240
Judo and karate	283
Rowing	180
Skating	180
Skiing:	
Moderate to steep	180
Downhill racing	367
Cross-country	270
Snowshoeing	187
Swimming:	
Pleasure	115
Freestyle—25–50 yards per minute	180
Butterfly—50 yards per minute	307
Backstroke—25–50 yards per minute	180
Breaststroke—25–50 yards per minute	180
Sidestroke—40 yards per minute	235
Volleyball	108
Waterskiing	163
Weight lifting	120
Wrestling	317
Yoga	60

WEEKLY PROGRESS SUMMARY CHART

Week _____ Weight at start _____ Waist at start _____

	Daily LifeSteps	75 Percent Portion Control Rule (Yes/No)			
		Breakfast	Lunch	Snack	Dinner
Monday	_____	_____	_____	_____	_____
Tuesday	_____	_____	_____	_____	_____
Wednesday	_____	_____	_____	_____	_____
Thursday	_____	_____	_____	_____	_____
Friday	_____	_____	_____	_____	_____
Saturday	_____	_____	_____	_____	_____
Sunday	_____	_____	_____	_____	_____
Total number of steps	_____	_____	_____	_____	_____
Average daily steps	_____	_____	_____	_____	_____

Weight at end of week _____

Waist at end of week _____

Weekly Progress Assessment (Please circle yes or no)

Achievement of Step Goal   Yes   No

Achievement of Portion Control Plan   Yes   No

Achievement of Weight-Loss Goal   Yes   No

Step Goal for Next Week: _____

they'll work a lot better if you help your kids get on track by setting a great example. That means that if you follow the Step Diet, it will be easier for them to follow it, too.

Remember, you are in charge. You can help your child with portion control, because

> ## PASSING THE TORCH
>
> Here's another motivator for overweight parents to reduce their own weight with the Step Diet: Their children are much more likely to become overweight than children of parents who aren't overweight. Don't just talk the talk—walk the walk!

you can control your own! You can help your child try foods that are filling but low in energy, because you can prepare and offer them. Research by Dr. Leann Birch at Penn State University has shown that kids who have been exposed to healthy foods are more likely to accept and incorporate them into their diets. Without this exposure early in life, it is unlikely kids will develop a preference for these foods as adults.

It is equally important for you to set a good example regarding physical activity. Get moving with your child—use every precious opportunity to walk and be active with your whole family. Instead of watching TV together, take a walk. Play with your children outside. If they see that you value physical activity, they will value it, too.

Small Changes for Small People

Children and adolescents can follow the Step Diet just as you follow it. Most kids will enjoy using step counters (you know how they love electronic gizmos). They will also enjoy setting personal goals (with your guidance) . . . and competing with you! Family members can set individual as well as family step goals and develop their own strategies for getting steps together as a family. Just as you listed ten ways for you to increase your steps, you can develop a list of ten ways for your entire family to increase their steps together.

Similarly, the strategy of not skipping meals and controlling portions at meals works very well with children. If your child is not already overweight, you don't need to use the 75 percent rule; just pay attention to portion size and passive overeating. You can also use the same sensible snacking rules that were discussed earlier in the book. Don't worry, your kids will get plenty to eat to support good growth, but you will reduce the likelihood of their overeating. If they are still hungry after finishing all their food, try to fill them up on healthier food options, including the free foods listed on pages 84–85.

One of the best ways to prevent your child from excess weight gain is to control the what, when, and how-much factors. Make sure *you're* in control, not them. Food is often too easily accessible, even to young children. Refrigerators and pantries stuffed with ready-to-eat or heat-and-eat foods make it too easy for kids to overeat the kind of things that should be eaten only in moderation. When mealtime rolls around, they are not hungry for the well-balanced meal you prepared. It's okay for them to eat a snack after school; just offer them a reasonable portion from among healthier items. Kids love cut-up fruit, for example—it is sweet, easy to eat, and full of good nutrition, yet it isn't loaded with calories.

What should you do about physical activity? Just as you did when you began the Step Diet, your child should begin by increasing his or her daily steps by 2,000. Kids are supposed to be more active than adults, so this is not excessive. Help them monitor their typical daily steps to determine a baseline. And be sure to check that your child is wearing the step counter every day, so it doesn't get lost or given away to a friend. You should also conduct a test run, as you did yourself, by counting out 100 steps and then making sure your child's step counter tallies up the same number.

Once you have established the baseline, instruct your child to add an additional 2,000 steps above this amount. You can jump-start this process by accompanying your child during a walk. Remember, when kids like something that gives them your attention, such as a walk together, they are likely to demand it frequently. It is impractical to think that your child all of a sudden will not want to watch TV, play video games, and send e-mail. The goal is to find a balance between sedentary time and active time.

What if Your Child Is Already Overweight?

If your child is currently overweight, should you use the 75 percent rule? First consult your pediatrician before attempting to put your child on any diet. However, the 75 percent rule can be effective with children and adolescents, since most of them are passively overeating just like their parents. Just make sure you use some common sense. Start by using the 75 percent rule at a few meals (maybe at dinner). If your child is still hungry after eating 75 percent, give him a little more. Make sure that you wait a few minutes before doing this, since it takes a while for our bodies to tell us we are full.

KIDS ARE NOT MINIATURE ADULTS

- Don't push it—kids get fatigued sooner than adults, so don't be rigid about "making quota" if your child seems overly tired during a walk. This could end up turning her off to the whole idea.

- Kids become overheated and dehydrated in a shorter time than adults do—make sure they get adequate liquids when on the move, especially on warmer days.

- Children get bored fast—so think of ways to divert them during a walk together. For example, try doing "silly walks" and having your child imitate you. Or have them guess how many steps it is from one place to another. Make a game of it!

We also recommend that you expose your children to lots of variety in foods—they are bound to like some of these foods, so experiment to find their favorites. Kids usually find small food items appealing—like baby carrots and mini muffins—so it's easy to help them manage portions and eat healthy at the same time.

As with the Step Diet for adults, it's important for overweight children to increase their physical activity. Simply counting LifeSteps works for kids, just as it does for adults. It will improve appetite control and, because it does not rely on strict food limitations to manage energy balance, gives your child the best chance of avoiding weight gain while still taking in plenty of energy for healthy growth.

On that note, how much activity is enough for a child? Because children are actively growing, their metabolism is constantly changing and increasing. So it is harder to set a step target based on resting energy expenditure and to make sure that 25 percent of total energy expenditure comes from physical activity. Children are inherently more active than adults. And younger kids are naturally more active than older kids. Therefore, your personal goal for steps as an adult may not be enough for your child.

Remember, young children are smaller than you and weigh less—so they use less energy than you when they move, and they don't go as far with each stride. Yet they don't eat vastly less than you. Thus, to keep from gaining excess weight, they need to get a lot more steps. We recommend that you try to increase your child's steps to at least 10,000, then see if you can increase this up to the 12,000 to 15,000 range. (For children over twelve years, shoot for at least 10,000 to 12,000 steps per day.) Do this gradually, adding 500 to 1,000 steps per week. Keep in mind that this will be less daunting for your child than for you, because kids are already more active than you at baseline and don't have as far to go to reach their goal. And remember to make it fun!

CHAPTER 6

A Body in Balance

Stage 5:
Find your
personal
energy
balance
point.

Congratulations! By now you have completed at least one twelve-week period of weight loss and have taken a major step toward your goal for weight management. You already have more knowledge than most diet plans leave you with, because you now know that energy balance is the secret to permanent weight control. "If you don't learn how to reestablish energy balance at your new reduced weight, you don't have much chance of keeping the weight off. That is why Stages 5 and 6 of the Step Diet are so important. You can't declare victory until you have shown you can keep the weight off. What you need to do now is find your *personal* balance between energy in and energy out—for life.

Monitor your weight and LifeSteps while learning to balance your MegaSteps.

Shift Your Focus

Many people who lose weight have trouble accepting the need to shift their focus from losing weight (creating negative energy balance) to keeping the weight off (maintaining energy balance). There is often an urge to try a little longer to lose some more. Again, we want to stress that losing weight is a "time-out" from real life that cannot be continued forever. Most people lose most of their weight during the first twelve weeks of a weight-loss plan. This is why we want you to stop losing weight now—regardless of how much weight you have lost.

At this point, you will likely be in one of two situations: (1) you have reached your weight-loss goal, or (2) you have lost weight but have not reached your goal, perhaps because your weight loss began to slow down or "plateau" before the end of twelve weeks, or because your goal is to lose more weight than you can achieve in one weight-loss cycle. Either way, it is time for you to take stock of where you are. If you have reached your weight goal, you may think you are done. In reality, no one is ever out of weight-gain danger in the environment we live in. We are surrounded by the temptation to eat and to sit, twenty-four hours a day, seven days a week. *Right now, you are at the point where most people fail.*

What If You Haven't Met Your Goal?

You have probably lost weight in your twelve weeks on the Step Diet, but perhaps not as much as you would have liked. You might have lost 20 pounds when your goal was to lose 50. Don't be discouraged! Twenty pounds kept off forever is a great accomplishment. Now, however, you need to be confident that you can maintain the degree of permanent behavior change that is necessary to keep the 20 pounds off before you even consider trying to lose more. The Step

Diet is designed to give you additional opportunities to lose weight, but you have to go through a complete cycle—setting a goal, losing weight, finding your personal balance to keep the weight off—before trying to lose any more weight.

You might ask, "Why can't I just keep going?" *Because that can set the stage for frustration and failure.* We don't want you to find that you can't maintain the behaviors needed to maintain a larger weight loss. Most people can't. If you can easily find your personal energy balance point to keep the 20 pounds off, you can go through another twelve-week weight-loss phase of the Step Diet. If you can't keep the first 20 pounds off, there is no reason to try to lose any more—you won't be able to maintain the behaviors necessary to maintain what you have lost, and you will just gain it all back. Twelve weeks is about the longest that most people can fully engage in losing weight.

If you haven't lost weight on the Step Diet, it's probably because you started it at a time when you couldn't make lifestyle changes a priority. Wait until you can before trying the Step Diet again.

Finding Your Personal Energy Balance

To stay at your new weight, you have to make sure that the energy you take in is the same as the energy your body burns. When thinking about your own energy balance, remember that there are only three big things that can change—your weight, how much you eat, and how much you move. Your genes are important, but these don't change. Your goal is to determine how much to eat and how much to move in order to keep your weight constant. How do you do this? Consider the figure on page 108.

Most diet plans focus almost totally on how much food you should eat and on calories. The problem is that of the three things you are most

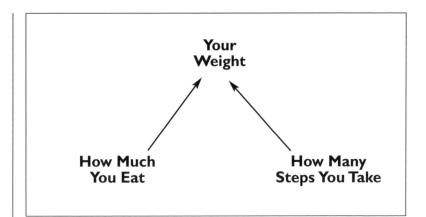

Your Weight

How Much You Eat

How Many Steps You Take

concerned about—weight, food intake, and physical activity—food intake (counting calories) is the hardest to measure accurately. The other two things—weight and physical activity—can be measured easily and accurately. The Step Diet focuses on monitoring those things that you can monitor accurately and easily—weight and steps—and adjusting food intake as needed. When you think about it in terms of energy balance, it seems pretty simple.

COUNTING CALORIES: AN INEXACT SCIENCE

In case you have a notion of keeping accurate track of your calories, think again. People are not good at it—it is just too hard to do in the real world. In fact, research has shown that people who keep diet diaries can misjudge the number of calories they eat by 25 to 30 percent. A better strategy for keeping your weight stable is to monitor your energy balance in steps (or MegaSteps), something you can actually measure. You can also measure your weight accurately, so that you can adjust your food intake down if your weight goes up.

Success Story 8

The 75 Percent Solution

Janet had lost 20 pounds on the Step Diet and had increased her daily LifeSteps to 11,000. Now her goal was to keep her weight off. But when she gained a couple of pounds, she found it difficult to walk more than 11,000 LifeSteps each day to burn more calories. So she simply used the 75 percent strategy at dinner. If this wasn't enough, she would use the strategy for other meals as well. Janet never counted calories—she just adjusted her portions based on her weight.

You Are Set for Success

If you have followed the Step Diet strategy to lose weight, you should be set up to keep off the weight you lost. Since you have compensated for your drop in metabolic rate (BodySteps) by increasing the steps you take each day (LifeSteps), your energy expenditure after weight loss should not be very different than your energy expenditure before weight loss. This is important because it means that you don't have to rely exclusively on food restriction to keep your weight off.

Now, you can't eat exactly the same number of calories you ate before weight loss, for two reasons. First, you were probably eating too much to begin with. Second, as you lost weight and your body got smaller, the number of steps it took to burn a calorie went up (it takes less energy to move a smaller body). Now you have to fine-tune your eating and physical activity to find your personal energy balance point.

Here is a simple strategy that will allow you to find your personal energy balance point.

• **Establish the maximum amount of physical activity that you can permanently incorporate into your daily life.** At a minimum, strive to take at least 10,000 LifeSteps each day and burn at least 25 percent of your daily energy expenditure through physical activity. Can you burn even more? Some people find they can get up to 15,000 to 20,000 steps a day, though most people find it difficult to get that many. Don't be afraid to set your sights high—the more physical activity you incorporate into your day, the less you have to worry about what you eat. Just develop a personal minimum daily step goal that's reasonable for you, and make sure you achieve that goal consistently. We all have days when it is harder to get our steps than others. For this reason, some people set a weekly goal for themselves by multiplying their daily goal by 7. The advantage of a weekly goal is that if you have trouble reaching your step goal on one day, you can make up for it on another day. Some people "bank" extra steps in anticipation of a day when they are not able to meet their step goal. You can have fun with these concepts, but make sure that, on average, you are meeting your daily LifeStep goal.

• **Make small adjustments to how much you eat in order to keep your body weight constant.** It is important to weigh yourself frequently so that you know when you need to adjust how much you eat. As you get comfortable with this technique, you will get better at adjusting how much you eat in order to keep your weight constant. If you find that you need to adjust your food intake, you might start by using the 75 percent strategy at dinner a few times each week. If this is not enough to stop weight gain, use the strategy at more meals. Remember to snack only if you are hungry and to snack sensibly. Focus on the free foods. They can satisfy your hunger without adding many calories.

• You can also make use of the tables in Appendix C on pages 236–270 to help ensure that the MegaStep value of the food you eat matches your body's total MegaStep energy expenditure. As you lose weight, the number of steps it takes you to burn 1 calorie goes up slightly. But don't worry if the MegaStep value for your total daily energy expenditure after weight loss is greater than the one you determined before weight loss—you will just use a different column in the tables in Appendix C (we will show you how). For example, before weight loss you might have had a total daily energy expenditure of 40 MegaSteps. After losing weight, your MegaStep total might go up to 52. This means that to maintain weight, you need to make sure that the energy value of the food you eat does not exceed 52 MegaSteps.

It Begins with Physical Activity

The first step in finding your personal energy balance point is maximizing the amount of physical activity you can maintain each and every day. When you started the Step Diet, you calculated your total energy expenditure in total steps per day (BodySteps plus LifeSteps), and you added LifeSteps during weight loss to compensate for the drop in your BodySteps as you lost weight. You also calculated the percentage of your total energy expenditure that was coming from physical activity. For most overweight people, this is less than 25 percent. To maximize your chances of being successful in keeping your weight off, you must have at least 25 percent of your total energy expenditure coming from physical activity and 75 percent or less coming from your resting metabolism. Now that you have lost weight, things have changed and you need to recalculate your energy expenditure in steps per day and to see if you have increased your LifeSteps to at least 25 percent of your total energy expenditure in steps per day.

Recalculate Your Total Energy Expenditure Following Weight Loss

Now that you have lost weight, it is necessary to recalculate your total energy expenditure. You will probably find it helpful to refer back to pages 69–70, where you calculated your total energy expenditure before weight loss.

1. Enter your pre–weight loss resting energy expenditure in BodySteps (you determined this in item 1 on page 69) here: _____ BodySteps/day.

2. Enter how many steps you needed to take to burn 1 calorie at your original body weight (you determined this on page 68). Write this starting steps per calorie value here: _____ steps/calorie.

3. Divide your pre–weight loss BodySteps per day value from item 1 above by your pre–weight loss steps/calorie value in item 2 to determine your starting resting metabolic rate in calories per day. Enter that value here: _____ calories per day.

4. To calculate the decline in your resting metabolism, multiply the number of pounds you lost by 8: I lost _____ pounds × 8 = _____ calories lost.

5. Subtract the calories lost determined in item 4 from your resting metabolism determined in item 3 to yield your new resting metabolism following weight loss in calories per day. Enter this value here: _____ calories per day after weight loss.

6. Use the table on pages 72–75 to determine how many steps you need to take to burn 1 calorie at your new body weight after weight loss. Enter that value here: _____ steps/calorie. This number should be larger than your steps/calorie value determined before weight loss.

7. Multiply the value you obtained in item 6 times the value you determined in item 5 to yield your new resting metabolic rate in BodySteps. Enter that value here: _____ BodySteps.

8. Record the average number of steps you get each day and that are measured on your step counter. Record your daily step value here: _____ steps/day.

9. Record the average number of steps you get each day from activities not measured by your step counter, such as swimming or biking. You can get the step equivalents for these activities on pages 98–99. Remember, this should be the average you get each day. Record this value here: _____ steps/day.

10. Add the numbers recorded in items 8 and 9 to get your total daily LifeSteps. Record that number here: _____ LifeSteps/day.

11. Add your total BodySteps (from item 7) and your LifeSteps (from item 10) to get your total daily steps. Record that value here: _____ total steps per day.

12. Divide your total daily steps by 1,000 to get your MegaSteps. Record that value here: _____. (Note: An easy way to do this without a calculator is to move the decimal point three places to the left—e.g., 41,000 steps becomes 41 MegaSteps). Round this to the nearest whole number to make it easy to remember.

13. Finally, determine the post–weight loss proportion of your total daily energy expenditure that comes from physical activity. To do this, divide your total LifeSteps (from item 10) by your total daily step (from item 11) and multiply by 100. Enter that value here: _____ percent of daily energy as physical activity.

HOW THIS FORMULA WORKS

Veronica is a twenty-five-year-old female who is 5 feet, 4 inches tall and weighed 185 pounds when she started the Step Diet. The number of steps she needed to take to burn 1 calorie at her starting weight was 19 (from the Steps per Calorie table on pages 72–75). Her previous estimated resting energy expenditure before weight loss was 32,138 BodySteps per day (from the BodySteps table in Appendix B on page 180). She lost 20 pounds with the Step Diet. Her average number of LifeSteps per day after weight loss was 12,000. The number of steps she needs to take to burn a calorie after weight loss is 22.

Let's see how Veronica calculated her new energy expenditure:

1. Veronica writes down her pre–weight loss resting energy expenditure in BodySteps: <u>32,138</u> BodySteps/day.

2. She then enters how many steps she needed to take to burn 1 calorie at her original body weight of 185 pounds: <u>19</u> steps/calorie.

3. She then divides her pre–weight loss BodySteps per day value from item 1 by her pre–weight loss steps/calorie value in item 2 to determine her starting resting metabolic rate in calories per day. She enters that value here: <u>1,691</u> calories per day.

4. To calculate the decline in her resting metabolism, she multiplies the number of pounds she lost by 8. She lost 20 pounds × 8 = <u>160</u> calories lost from her resting metabolism.

5. She subtracts the calories lost determined in item 4 from her resting metabolism determined in item 3 to yield her new resting metabolism following weight loss in calories per day. She enters this value here: <u>1,531</u> calories per day after weight loss.

6. Veronica enters the number of steps she needs to take to burn 1 calorie at her new body weight after weight loss: <u>22</u> steps/calorie.

7. She multiplies the value obtained in item 6 times the value determined in item 5 to yield her new resting metabolic rate in Body-Steps. She enters that value here: <u>33,682</u> BodySteps.

8. Next, she records the average number of steps she gets each day and that are measured on her step counter: <u>12,000</u> steps/day.

9. She then records the average number of steps she gets each day from activities not measured by her step counter, such as swimming or biking: <u>0</u> steps/day.

10. Veronica adds the numbers recorded in items 8 and 9 to get her total daily LifeSteps and records the number here: <u>12,000</u> LifeSteps/day.

11. She then adds her total BodySteps (from item 7) and her LifeSteps (from item 10) to get her total daily steps: <u>45,682</u> total steps per day.

12. Veronica rounds up her total daily steps to 46,000 and divides by 1,000 to get MegaSteps. She then records the value: <u>46</u> .

13. Finally, Veronica determines the post–weight loss proportion of her total daily energy expenditure that comes from physical activity. To do this, she divides her total LifeSteps (from item 10) by her total daily steps (from item 11) and multiplies by 100. This yields a value of: <u>26.3</u> percent of daily energy as physical activity.

Finding the Right Balance

If the portion of your total energy expenditure from physical activity is less than 25 percent, you should try to increase your physical activity. First, you can look for ways to get more steps during the day. (Review the list on pages 37–42.) In addition, you should consider setting aside some time each day for planned physical activity. This can be a planned walk or a bike ride or a swim. Be adventurous. Consider joining a sports team or taking up an activity, such as tennis or golf, that you can play throughout your life. Try mountain biking, mountain climbing, or canoeing. You're sure to find something you enjoy that enriches your life.

Think about your day from the time you wake up to the time you go to bed. Where are the opportunities for more steps? Can you get up fifteen minutes earlier to walk? How about ten? Can you walk fifteen minutes before you go to bed? If you go through your day hour by hour, you will likely find some times and places for more steps.

Think about your typical day and identify possible times for more activity. In the spaces provided, write down the times during your typical day that you might be able to add more LifeSteps, and list the activities you could do to increase your steps.

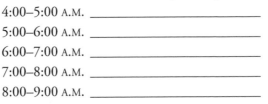

SUCCESS TIP

Pick a Time to Walk When the Time Is Right

Many people find it easier to stick with a daily routine for walking, whether it's early in the morning, at midday, or in the evening. The key here is consistency, not when you do it. You're more likely to stick with your physical activity if it's part of a predictable pattern rather than something you fit into random pockets of time. Simply find a time that you can devote to physical activity each day.

4:00–5:00 A.M. _____

5:00–6:00 A.M. _____

6:00–7:00 A.M. _____

7:00–8:00 A.M. _____

8:00–9:00 A.M. _____

9:00–10:00 A.M. _____

10:00–11:00 A.M. _____

11:00 A.M.–12:00 P.M. _____

12:00–1:00 P.M. _____

1:00–2:00 P.M. _____

2:00–3:00 P.M. _____

3:00–4:00 P.M. _____

4:00–5:00 P.M. _____

5:00–6:00 P.M. _____

6:00–7:00 P.M. _____

7:00–8:00 P.M. _____

8:00–9:00 P.M. _____

9:00–10:00 P.M. _____

10:00–11:00 P.M. _____

11:00 P.M.–12:00 A.M. _____

Rain or Sleet or Snow or Hail . . .

The weather will not always cooperate with your plans to add thousands of steps to your daily output. What do you do then?

• **The mall.** Today's supersized malls provide plenty of territory for walking, with enough visual diversions en route to keep you from getting bored. And don't forget the fringe benefit: You can pick up a few things you've been meaning to buy while you're there.

• **Office stairwells.** Use the stairs in your office or apartment building to log some extra steps.

• **A treadmill.** An indoor treadmill provides a convenient way to get steps in at any time. Manual ones are cheaper (under $200), but the more expensive electrical ones are far superior and provide a more pleasant and consistent walking experience. Be sure to get one that has good stability and smooth belt action.

• **Aqua jogging.** Walking in the water is a refreshing way to add steps (although you won't be able to wear your step counter in the pool). Of course, you can swim there too, for a great workout (see the conversion table with step equivalents for swimming on pages 98–99).

Maintaining Your Step Goal

You should now have a personal minimum LifeStep goal for weight maintenance. It is important that you monitor your physical activity regularly to make sure that you achieve this goal on a consistent basis. For some of you, your step counter has become part of your daily life, and monitoring your daily steps is second nature.

Success Story 9

Faster Commute Creates Time Slot for Walking

Andi had a long drive to work every day and spent most of her workday in meetings or at her computer. She was so tired when she got home at night that it was hard to get motivated to go for a walk. A co-worker told her that if she left for work a half hour later in the morning, traffic would be a lot lighter, and she could still get to work at the same time. So Andi began leaving home a half hour later, and she used the extra time at home to walk on the treadmill. The new routine helped get her weight under control and gave her more energy at work.

We highly recommend wearing your step counter all the time. But if you don't wear it every day, at least use it periodically to ensure that you are achieving your minimum step goal. You may want to wear your step counter more frequently at first (for example, for a week every month or every other month), just to make sure you are accomplishing your goal. As you get more comfortable keeping your weight off, you can monitor your steps less frequently.

It can also be beneficial to write down the number of steps you take periodically. Scientific research from the National Weight Control Registry and from Drs. Tom Wadden and Gary Foster at the University of Pennsylvania suggests that record keeping is a marker of success in weight management. We recommend that, every month or so, you write down the number of LifeSteps you take each day for a week. If you are meeting your minimum step goals, you will be reassured. If not, this will be a wake-up call for making sure you get your physical activity back on track.

Making Small Adjustments in How Much You Eat

Although you have been eating 75 percent of your food and losing weight, you may have found that your weight loss slowed or even stopped by the end of the twelve-week period. If this was the case for you, the amount of food you have been eating is about what you will need to continue eating to maintain your weight. If you continued to lose weight throughout the entire twelve-week weight-loss period, you may be able to relax the

SUCCESS TIP

Talk About Taking Household Chores to the Next Step!

• Add in extra trips to the washing machine by taking only half a basket of clothes each time.

• Why make one trip to the mailbox when you can make two or three? Divide up that pile of bill payments and log some extra trips.

• This one's a no-brainer. Add another lap around the block when you take Bowser out for his daily strolls.

75 percent rule a little bit at this point. This is because you no longer want to be in negative energy balance, and your increase in physical activity alone is enough to maintain your weight. Based on your new situation, let's review your options meal by meal throughout the day.

• **Breakfast.** This is the best meal-time to experiment with relaxing your 75 percent strategy. Research has shown that you get filled up more easily with food you eat in the morning as compared to food you eat in the evening. You are much more likely to overeat later in the day than at breakfast.

• **Lunch.** If you are still hungry and you are not gaining weight, you can relax your 75 percent rule at lunch and see what happens. If you start gaining weight, go back to the 75 percent rule.

• **Dinner and snacks.** These are the last meals for which you should try to relax the 75 percent rule, because they often present bigger challenges. You might start by relaxing the rule every other day and see how it goes. If you get into trouble, you can always go back to the 75 percent strategy for all meals and snacks.

Many of you will find that eating 75 percent of your food does not represent food restriction for you. However, if you feel that you have been eating less than what you need to fill you up, it's time to relax the 75 percent rule.

You may find, over time, that you will start serving yourself smaller portions that are actually equivalent to 75 percent of what you used to eat. This is okay, and it just means that your food portion "IQ" has gone way up, and you know what a reasonable portion looks like. However, if your weight starts to creep up, go back to being more careful about eating only 75 percent of what is served.

It is possible (but not likely) that some of you may gain weight when you eat 75 percent of your food. If this is the case, you have only two options. First, you can increase your physical activity even more. This is the best solution. However, if you find that you just cannot increase your physical activity any more, you have to eat even less. For example, you might try eating 50 percent of one meal each day and 75 percent of your other meals. Experiment, but keep it simple. And make sure the change is something you can do permanently.

The MegaSteps Energy Balance Method

Now that you have reached your personal energy balance point, you might benefit from occasionally monitoring your energy balance. As we have said before, it is almost impossible to do this by counting calories in the food you eat and in your physical activity, but you can do this pretty accurately by monitoring your MegaSteps. On pages 112–13 you recalculated your energy expenditure in MegaSteps after weight loss. One of your simple goals for weight maintenance is to make sure that

TURN DEAD TIME INTO ACTIVE TIME

You can get extra LifeSteps during the day—even when you're doing something else:

- Try walking around the house while you're scanning the front page, checking the latest stats on your favorite teams, or flipping through catalogs.

- Use a cordless phone when having long conversations, and walk while you talk.

- Instead of channel surfing during commercials, put the remote down and do some "surfing" yourself. Take a walk around the house and get some air during those breaks. Some people walk on a treadmill while they watch TV.

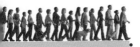

you achieve this MegaStep goal every day. Now you can also use the food tables in Appendix C to calculate the MegaStep value of your diet. This is a simple, fun way to check that you are in energy balance.

To use the MegaStep Energy Balance method, you have to know how many steps it takes you to burn 1 calorie—called your step per calorie value. You wrote this on page 68, and then revised it on page 112. To use the tables in Appendix C, find the column that corresponds to your steps per calorie value. Then just add up the MegaStep value of the foods you eat in a day. If you are in energy balance, it should be very close to the MegaStep value of your daily energy expenditure. Remember, if you eat more MegaSteps of food than you burn, you will gain weight. If you eat fewer MegaSteps than you burn, you will lose weight.

For example, Jennifer burns 35 MegaSteps each day. For a week, she wrote down all the foods she ate. She then used Appendix C to find the MegaStep value for all of these foods. Jennifer used the third column of the tables, since she determined on page 70 that she gets 23 steps per calorie. She found that on average, the MegaStep value of her food was 34 MegaSteps per day. Jennifer felt comfortable that she was in energy balance.

Ashley used the tables in Appendix C to experiment with new foods to add to her weight-maintenance diet. She gets 41 MegaSteps per day and designed some menus that added up to 41 MegaSteps per day. In this way, Ashley learned how to incorporate new foods into her life without worrying that she was not maintaining energy balance.

"Buying" an Occasional Fun Food

Most people who lose weight manage to keep it off for a while, but it gradually comes back. Generally, this happens when people get tired of the restrictive nature of their weight plan and miss their favorite foods. Would you be happy if you had to go without your favorite dessert forever? When you understand energy balance and begin using your energy balance skills, you can enjoy all kinds of foods without worrying about gaining weight back. It is just like deciding to treat yourself to a vacation at the beach. Yes, you could get by without it, but it's fun! Sure, it costs extra money, but you can plan for this by saving ahead or paying it off over time. You can incorporate your fun foods into your diet in a similar manner.

Using the MegaStep Energy Balance method, you can incorporate some of your favorite fun foods into your diet. You can do this in a couple of ways. First, you can find the MegaStep value of the food you want to add

Q. I don't feel like I have increased my portion sizes by very much, yet my weight is creeping up. I am really frustrated!

A. Your weight may be creeping up for a couple of reasons. For one, your energy needs have dropped with weight loss, so your body does not require as much energy as before. Make sure you use the calculations on pages 112–13 to estimate how much your resting energy expenditure (BodySteps) has dropped. In order to keep your new weight, use the tables in Appendix C to make sure that the foods you eat do not total more than your total daily energy expenditure in MegaSteps. Even if you are increasing portion sizes only a little, you may still be taking in too much energy in the foods you eat. Second, it is very easy to underestimate your portion sizes. Go back to Chapter 1 and look at some of the tools for determining portion size, to make sure that you are not a victim of "portion distortion."

and take this amount of MegaSteps away from the rest of your diet. In other words, just eat less of other things. Another way to incorporate an occasional fun food into your diet is to add extra LifeSteps to your day. This will increase your MegaStep total for the day and you can add this food to what you are already eating. So, if you want to add a chocolate fudge ice cream from Baskin-Robbins, and you get 21 steps per calorie (column 3 of the tables in Appendix C), you need to add an extra 7 MegaSteps (7,000 LifeSteps) to afford this luxury. You might work hard to get an extra 1,000 LifeSteps each day for a week and treat yourself to the ice cream on Sunday.

If, instead of giving yourself an extra treat, you want to take a day off from step counting, you can also save extra steps to trade for sedentary time using the MegaStep Energy Balance method. For example, if you want to spend an entire day being inactive, you can use the extra LifeSteps you walked another day to achieve that day's LifeStep goal, and take a day off.

Eight Principles of Weight-Loss Maintenance

If you cannot maintain the changes you have made, you will gain back the weight you have lost. How frustrating and discouraging! To help you on your way, we'd like you to consider eight principles of perma-nent weight management that we've learned from years of study. Some of these points have already been dis-cussed, but they are so important that they are worth repeating.

IT GETS BETTER

Participants in the National Weight Control Registry tell us that it gets easier over time to keep weight off. Also, physical activity becomes some-thing that is important and enjoyable.

principle 1 You must find your own personal level of energy balance to keep weight off. You alone will decide how much of your behavior change will come from eating fewer calories and how much will come from increasing the energy you burn in physical activity. Unlike other diets, this is not a one-size-fits-all prescription. Your energy balance point is unique to you and within your control. We will help you to determine your new personal energy balance point so that you can maintain your weight loss. Try the MegaStep Energy Balance method to check that you are in energy balance and to safely experiment with adding new foods to your diet.

principle 2 Increasing physical activity improves your chances of keeping weight off. The evidence clearly demonstrates that you are not likely to succeed in achieving energy balance at low levels of energy intake and energy expenditure. This strategy requires permanent and significant food restriction, a behavior that is very hard to sustain. The more physical activity you can incorporate consistently into your lifestyle, the less you will have to rely on food restriction or unusual food choices to keep your weight off. Physical activity improves appetite control and makes unintentional overeating less likely. It also has great psychological benefits. Most people we talk to who engage in daily physical activity describe it as a stress reliever, a pleasant way to spend time alone or with friends, a way to take stock of their life and their priorities. It improves their mood and gives them a better outlook on life.

principle 3 Losing weight is temporary, but keeping weight off requires a lifestyle that you can live with permanently. We explained previously that your resting metabolic rate—the rate at which your body burns energy at rest—actually goes down as you lose weight. After weight loss, there is less of you, and a smaller body needs less energy. Because you now need less energy, you cannot go back to the same old lifestyle, or you will surely gain the weight back. It is critical that you find a new lifestyle that you can live with for the rest of your life.

principle 4 **If you were overweight before, you are at high risk of becoming overweight again— and you must make avoiding weight gain a high priority.** Successful participants in the National Weight Control Registry tell us that keeping their weight off is a constant concern—not an obsession, but a lifelong focus. They don't complain, because they all tell us that life is much better after weight loss. That's why they pay attention to their weight and put weight maintenance high on their list of life priorities. The more you can build the key behaviors for weight maintenance into your daily routine, the better your chances for long-term success.

principle 5 **You must plan for events that produce stress.** Most people tend to relax their vigilance about eating and physical activity during stressful times. If you don't want to regain your weight—particularly during the first six to twelve months after you've lost it—you need to plan for those days of "personal disaster" that befall all of us. You might find that you can use physical activity to manage your stress. You might try yoga or meditation. Whatever you do, don't turn to food. It may look comforting, but overindulging will make you feel out of control. Many people find it helpful to put more structure into their eating and physical activity patterns during times of stress. You may want to return to the 75 percent rule for all foods during high-stress periods. Making a list of your own personal strategies for dealing with stress will help.

Strategies that I will implement when stressed:

1. _____

2. _____

3. _____

principle 6   **You have to weigh yourself regularly.** How are you going to know if you are maintaining your new weight unless you weigh yourself regularly? Don't obsess over your weight and start getting on the scale five times a day. Once or twice per week will do. If you consistently begin weighing 3 to 5 or more pounds heavier, you are likely regaining weight and should examine your behaviors to assess the possible causes of the positive energy balance.

Remember, your bathroom scale and your step counter are the two best tools you have to manage your weight. If your weight is going up, you must be eating more, taking fewer steps, or both—that is the only

Success Story 10
Making Room for Dessert

Charlene loves banana splits, but they obviously do not fit into her weight-control plan. In order to enjoy a banana split every now and then—without feeling guilty or gaining weight—Charlene uses the MegaSteps Energy Balance method to "save up" for her favorite treat. Using the tables in Appendix C, she found that a McDonald's hot fudge sundae is 8 MegaSteps. She decided to save up for one week preparing for this treat. She ate 1 Mega-Step less each day for a week (saving 7 MegaSteps) and added 200 LifeSteps per day over the week (an additional 1.4 Mega-Steps). By eating a little less and moving a little more, she saved up 8.4 MegaSteps—more than enough for the hot fudge sundae.

way you could be in positive energy balance. Your step counter will tell you if your LifeSteps have declined from the level you determined was necessary to maintain your weight. If your LifeSteps have remained constant at your goal and you are still gaining, then your food energy intake must have increased. Then you will need to examine your food intake pattern and make sure you are continuing to eat 75 percent of your food. Also, use the tables in Appendix C to make sure that your food intake in MegaSteps is equal to or less than your MegaStep energy expenditure that you determined on pages 112–13 after weight loss.

Success Story 11

Extra Pregame Steps Prevent Postgame Letdown

Bobby was looking forward to spending New Year's Day watching football with his friends. How was he going to get in his 11,000 steps? Sure, he could take a couple of walks to squeeze in some steps, but not 11,000. There were too many good games to watch! Bobby decided that he would save up for some sedentary time. For a week before the big day, he banked an extra 1,000 steps each day. It wasn't easy going from 11,000 to 12,000 steps, but he was pretty motivated. By New Year's Day, he had an extra 7,000 steps in the bank. Now he just had to get in 4,000 steps that day, which he did by convincing his friends to throw a football around at halftime during one of the games. Bobby had a great time watching football, with no penalty for being sedentary on game day.

principle 7

Start every day with breakfast. Most participants in the National Weight Control Registry eat breakfast every single day, and research is mounting to suggest that people who eat breakfast eat less during the rest of the day.

principle 8

Seek balance in all aspects of your life. Successful weight maintainers have found a balance not just between energy intake and expenditure, but also in their physical, mental, emotional, and spiritual lives. Because behavior change is hard to maintain, the more you can link desired new behaviors with other essential aspects of your life, the more likely you are to succeed. For example, if your walking (or swimming, or time on the treadmill) enhances your well-being, you will be more likely to stick with it.

What if I Regain Weight?

Some of you may find that some or all of the weight you lost comes back. Perhaps your life circumstances have changed and you are no longer able to meet your step goal. If this happens to you, it is okay to try the Step Diet again. But first figure out why you were unable to maintain the lifestyle changes you made. If you do the same thing a second time, you will most likely regain the weight. Try to problem-solve. What did you do right? What did you do wrong?

It is likely that *all* of you will have some occasions where you fail to follow your weight-management plan. Perhaps you go for a few days

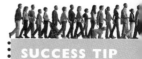

SUCCESS TIP

Periods of stress make it easy to indulge in behaviors that are not within the boundaries of your Step Diet. If you are concerned about gaining weight during periods of stress:

• Log your LifeSteps during this period to make sure you are meeting your physical activity goals.

• Go back to using the 75 percent rule for all of your food until the stressful period is over.

• Make sure you have healthy snacks available.

• Find some time for yourself each day.

without meeting your step goal or perhaps overdo it on the intake side for a few days. These are slips that everyone has. The main thing is not to let a slip become a relapse during which you regain all of your weight. You need to get back on track either by losing the weight again or making sure you don't gain any more.

We find that some people who encounter a slip convince themselves that they have "blown it," and a slip becomes a relapse. Don't let this happen to you. You have worked too hard to get where you are.

TIPS FOR WEIGHING YOURSELF

• **If you choose to weigh yourself weekly, pick the same day each week.** Some people like to weigh themselves daily, given that it is easy to build into a routine. However, due to normal body fluid fluctuations, it is normal for your weight to vary by as much as 3 to 5 pounds per day. Therefore, the best way to see if you are holding, gaining, or losing weight is to record your weight once per week.

• **Weigh yourself at the same time of day.** Weighing yourself first thing in the morning without clothes on will give you the best measurement of your weight.

• **Use the same scale.** If you have more than one scale in your home, use just one. Scales fluctuate and often read differently.

• **Remain positive, whether or not you have lost weight.** Pounds on the scale are only one indicator of whether or not you are losing body fat, a better indicator of overall health status. Remember the other ways to measure your success: waist circumference, how many steps you are walking each day, and your overall sense of well-being.

CHAPTER 7

Keep the Weight Off . . . Forever

The more you know about energy balance, the more likely that you will be successful in keeping your weight off. Think of this chapter as a graduate seminar in energy balance—information for the more serious student of weight management. If you're eager to learn about starting another cycle of weight loss, turn to Chapter 8. If you're in less of a hurry, read on.

By now, you should know that what happens to your weight is a direct consequence of your state of

Stage 6:
Plan for lifelong success.

Refine your energy balance skills.

energy balance, and that the only way to lose weight is through negative energy balance. Since you've already lost weight, your goal now is an energy balance that maintains your weight. This seems simple, but a major barrier to this goal is that you have no easy way to know your state of energy balance in the short term, other than the bathroom scale. You can be eating 5 to 10 MegaSteps more per day than you burn, and you might not realize this for several days, until your weight creeps up. You have never before had a feasible way to monitor your state of energy balance. As we've discussed, the MegaStep Energy Balance method is a fun, easy way to keep track of your energy balance.

And now you can learn how to maximize the number of MegaSteps you burn each day.

Your Body Is Like Your Car

When you eat, you consume proteins, carbohydrates, fats—even alcohol. These are called *macronutrients*. When your body burns these substances, energy (calories) is released. This energy can be used for fuel to meet the body's immediate needs, or it can be stored to provide energy for future needs. If you don't ingest as much energy as you burn in a day, you have to get fuel from stored energy (body fat). This is very similar to your car's use of gasoline. Think of your body fat as the amount of gas in your gas tank. Your energy expenditure is the amount of gas your car uses in a day, and your energy intake is the amount of gas you put into your tank each day. Let's say that you drive a distance that burns ten gallons of gasoline in a day. If you put in ten gallons of gas over the day, the amount of gas in your tank will be the same at the beginning and end of the day. If you put in only five gallons of gas, your car will burn those five gallons plus another five gallons that are stored in your gas tank. The amount of gas in your tank goes down. If, alternatively, you put in fifteen gallons of gas during the day and burn ten, you will have an extra five gallons of gas. Your body fat is also a place to store extra energy. The problem is, many people have too much extra energy.

> ## MYTH: FAT AND CARBOHYDRATE BLOCKERS CAN HELP YOU LOSE WEIGHT
>
> Some weight-loss products claim to help you lose weight by blocking your absorption of fat or carbohydrates. While there are some drugs (such as Orlistat) that do this, over-the-counter products are not likely to be beneficial for weight management.

Rather than use our stored fuel, we just keep adding gas to our tank—because we constantly take in more energy than we burn. Unlike your gas tank, your body fat stores never become full. They just keep expanding to hold the extra energy.

How can you affect the way your car converts gasoline into energy? Can you change the type of gasoline you use? Can you do anything to help your car burn gasoline more or less efficiently? We can ask these same questions about your body. Can you change the type of food you eat to affect how your body converts food to energy? Can you do anything to help your body convert food to energy more or less efficiently?

Most fad diet books suggest that some macronutrients are better or worse for weight loss than others. Depending on the book, for example, carbs can be bad guys or good guys. Others suggest that if you eat only monounsaturated fats or low-glycemic foods, you will lose weight easily. The truth is that different macronutrients are converted into fuel differently by the body, but the importance of these differences for energy balance is very small. Energy balance is mostly about energy in versus energy out. Still, it can be useful to know a little about how the macronutrients differ and how these differences affect energy balance.

Energy Density

Different macronutrients provide a different number of calories per gram (the metric unit for weight), which means they have different energy densities. Energy density is the amount of energy (typically given in calories) per unit weight of food. Why is this important? Because the energy density of a diet may affect how much food you eat. Some research suggests that you eat more total energy when the foods you eat are high in energy density. If your diet is high in fat, for example, it is likely to be higher in energy density than a diet high in carbohydrates or protein. This is one reason that many weight-management experts advocate a low-fat diet; it may help you avoid overeating.

The energy density of your diet is determined not just by the macronutrients in the foods you eat but also by the things in your

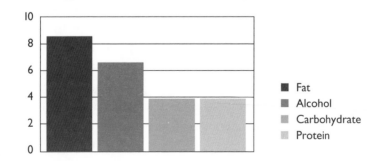

Energy Density of Macronutrients (Calories per Gram)

■ Fat
■ Alcohol
■ Carbohydrate
■ Protein

foods that do not provide energy, such as fiber and
water. The more fiber and water in a food, the lower
its energy density. Thus, most fruits and vegetables
have low energy densities compared to fast foods,
snacks, and desserts. Your diet's energy density can
affect how many total calories (and MegaSteps) you
eat. In the short term, people eat more total calories
with a high-energy-density diet than with a low-
energy-density diet. There are no long-term data
relating energy density to body weight gain or weight
maintenance, but it is likely that lowering the energy
density of your diet can help in weight maintenance.
In this way, energy density may have an impact on
energy balance as well.

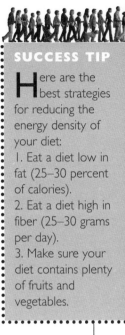

Most foods that are inherently low in energy are
high in water and fiber and low in fat. Most vegetables
fall into this category and are routinely stigmatized as
"diet foods." If you like vegetables, this is great; you can eat pretty
much all you want without gaining weight. If you don't like vegetables,
then you should try to identify as many foods as you can that are low
in calories for their weight. Such foods would be characterized as being
low in energy density. Many studies have shown that foods low in
energy density fill you up faster and reduce the probability that you
will eat too many calories and gain weight. The free foods listed on pages
84–85 are low-energy-density foods. It would be hard to eat enough
of these foods to cause weight gain.

Go out and explore! With most big grocery stores offering some
10,000 to 50,000 different food items, you are bound to find numerous
foods you like that have relatively low energy density and could become
important items in your weight-management menu.

THE ATKINS DIET RAGE

Currently, high-protein, low-carbohydrate diets, such as Atkins and South Beach, are popular. James Hill was an author of a recent study published in the *New England Journal of Medicine* that evaluated a low-carb diet as compared to a low-fat diet. While a low-carbohydrate diet produced greater weight loss than a low-fat diet at three and six months, there was no difference in weight loss between the diets at one year. In fact, most people on both diets either dropped out or kept off very little weight. It emphasizes that popular diets are focused more on helping you lose weight than on helping you keep it off.

The table below groups foods into different categories of energy density. You should try to choose more foods from the low and very low energy-density categories and limit your intake of foods from the medium and high categories. (A quick way to determine a food's energy density is to divide the calories in a serving by the grams in a serving, as noted on the nutrition label. You will end up with the number of calories per gram.)

Within each macronutrient category, you have choices about the types of nutrients you consume. You can, for example, choose between many different sources of protein, carbohydrates, and fat. There is a

Energy Density	Calorie Density	Foods
Very low	Fewer than 0.6 calories per gram	Fruits, vegetables, soups
Low	0.6–1.5 calories per gram	Lean meat, starches, fruits and vegetables, beans
Medium	1.5–4.0 calories per gram	Cheese, salad dressings, some snack foods, desserts
High	4.0–9.0	Chocolate, nuts, chips, deep-fried foods, candy

great deal of popular interest in consuming more healthy forms of carbohydrates and fat, although the experts do not agree about what constitutes "healthiest." Current recommendations emphasize whole grains as desirable sources of carbohydrates while simultaneously favoring a balanced fat intake that consists of monounsaturated fats (such as olive oil and vegetable oil—soybean oil, corn oil, sunflower oil) and a limited intake of saturated fats (such as butter, lard, tallow) and trans fats (such as shortening and margarine).

Are There Good and Bad Fats?

You may have heard advice to eat more foods containing polyunsaturated fats, monounsaturated fats, and even fish oils, and fewer foods containing saturated fats or trans fats. This will probably improve your overall health by improving your lipid profile (lowering bad cholesterol), and it might reduce your risk of developing heart disease. But changing types of fat will not affect your energy balance or your weight management. You will not magically lose weight or have an easier time maintaining your weight loss. All types of fats provide 9 calories per gram consumed. The point is that managing your body weight is about balancing total energy in with total energy out.

SUCCESS TIP

Reducing the energy density of your diet may help you better manage your food intake.

Are There Good and Bad Carbs?

You might have heard that carbohydrates from fruit and vegetable sources may be better for you than carbohydrates coming from foods containing a lot of refined sugar. No big surprise. Just as all fats are not bad, all carbohydrates are not bad. The current public perception is that carbs are bad (a few years ago, it was that fats are bad), and many dieters

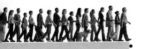

are trying to avoid all carbohydrates to lose weight. This is not a very good strategy, since carbohydrates are important sources of key nutrients for the body. A more reasonable strategy is to try to eat carbohydrates from fruits, vegetables, and whole, natural grains and limit intake of refined carbohydrates.

But will eating more fruits and vegetables help you lose weight or keep your weight off? Scientists are still not clear about the answer to this question. No research studies clearly show that eating a diet high in fruits and vegetables helps with weight loss. However, a diet high in fruits and vegetables tends to be low in energy density, so it makes sense that it may help you manage energy intake better.

Some diet books recommend that you choose low-glycemic carbohydrates. The glycemic index of a food is the extent to which your blood sugar increases after you eat that food. In general, foods containing simple sugars have a high glycemic index (they cause a rapid increase in blood sugar), while those containing complex carbohydrates (such as whole grains) have a low glycemic index. Some people think that foods that make your blood sugar rise rapidly (high-glycemic-index foods) cause weight gain. Most scientists are not convinced that the glycemic index of a food directly affects body weight, but this may change as more research is done. It does make sense to avoid excessive amounts of simple sugars and to go for more complex carbohydrates like whole grains.

What About Reduced-Calorie Foods and Artificial Sweeteners?

We are bombarded like never before with a wide array of calorie-modified foods: low-calorie, low-fat, low-carb, low-glycemic-index. These foods can help in weight management, but only if they are used the right way. Critics of such foods point out that people who use them may end up eating more ("I ate the whole box because it said they were low-fat") and may get more total energy intake than if they ate the full-calorie version of the food. But let's give ourselves more credit than that. If you use your head, these reduced-calorie foods can be great tools for your weight management.

Artificial sweeteners are also great options that allow you to enjoy a sweet taste without guilt. The available evidence suggests that these products do help with weight management and are used by successful weight maintainers. If a diet soda provides the "fun" of a soft drink without the extra energy, go for it. As for safety, artificial sweeteners have been carefully evaluated and approved by the U.S. Food & Drug Administration, the agency that is charged with protecting the safety of our food supply. Some people object to consuming products that they do not think are natural, and that is a matter of personal choice. The best data we now have suggest that artificial sweeteners can be useful in weight management.

Don't Forget to Count Alcohol

Protein, carbohydrates, and fat are the main energy-contributing components of our diets, but alcohol is also energy dense—about 7 calories per gram. It is also similar to fat in the amount of energy it provides, something many people don't realize. A 6-ounce glass of wine has 125 calories—1.3–4.8 MegaSteps, depending on your body size—almost twice that of a similar amount of soda. Don't deprive yourself if you enjoy a drink now and then, but if you regularly consume alcohol, cutting back a bit can save hundreds of calories in just a few days. Cutting out all alcohol may be too big a change. You can do it for a while but not forever. Cutting back just a little saves calories and may be a change you can live with for good.

Your Body's Calorie-Burning Ability

Your body is constantly burning energy, even while you sleep. Burning protein, carbohydrates, and fat provides energy your body needs to keep your heart beating and your blood pumping, to make hormones, and to sustain many other functions that keep you alive. The entire amount of energy your body burns is called your total energy expenditure (or total metabolism), and it is composed of three main components.

1. Resting Metabolic Rate (RMR)

Your RMR, as we discussed earlier, is the amount of energy your body burns at rest. In a medical setting, this is often measured while you sleep or lie quietly. In most people, it is the single largest component of total daily energy expenditure. It is directly related to your body size and proportional to the amount of your body that is not fat—your so-called fat-free mass, most of which is muscle and bone. The bigger you are, the more fuel you burn, in the same way that a big house needs a bigger furnace than a small house. When you gain weight, you burn more fuel to keep your body working, and when you lose weight, your body burns less fuel.

Your resting metabolic rate is largely determined by your body size: Larger people burn more energy during the day than smaller people. It also varies a little depending on your sex (it's higher in men because of more muscle mass) and your age (it goes down with age because of declining muscle mass). If you turn to the tables on pages 180–235, finding your sex, your body weight, your height, and your age will give you your estimated daily resting metabolic rate in terms of BodySteps.

Many people believe that if they are overweight or obese, they burn less energy than a lean person does. This is true if you consider the amount of energy burned per pound of body weight. Because lean people have a greater proportion of body weight that is muscle, as well as less fat, they will burn more energy per pound of body weight. Overweight or obese people actually burn more total energy (and BodySteps) per day at rest, however, because they are significantly larger. For example, a forty-five-year-old lean woman who is 5 feet, 5 inches tall and weighs 120 pounds would have a resting metabolic rate of about 1,281 calories per day. This means that she burns about 10 calories per pound of body weight. A woman who is the same height but weighs 180 pounds would have a resting metabolic rate of about 1,541 calories per day. Thus, her resting metabolic rate is greater than the lean woman's, but the energy she burns per pound of body weight (about 8.5 calories per pound) is less. So, in practical terms, the overweight woman must eat more total energy each day to maintain her weight. No matter what you might have heard to the contrary, this is the scientific truth.

When you lose weight, your resting metabolic rate *will* go down. You will have become a lighter person, so you will burn less energy at rest—this is an incontrovertible fact. There is very little you can do to prevent a drop in your resting metabolic rate. That's the bad news. The good news is that you can make up for the drop in your resting metabolism that occurs with weight loss by increasing your voluntary energy expenditure (LifeSteps)—that is, engaging in a simple physical activity, like walking.

We have studied hundreds of people during weight loss and found that resting metabolism drops by about 8 calories for each pound of weight lost. So, if you lose 10 pounds, you will burn 80 fewer calories in a day from then on, provided you stay at that weight. If you lose 30 pounds, you will lose 240 calories of expenditure, and so on. This is why most people are unable to maintain weight loss. They lose the weight and then go back to the same lifestyle they had before they went on the diet. If they wanted to maintain the weight loss permanently—without doing any more physical activity (for example, through modifying food intake *only*)—they would have to eat at least 240 calories (2.4–9.1 MegaSteps, depending on body size) less per day, every day. A life sentence of reduced intake, without parole!

Obviously, your weight-management efforts would be helped if your RMR were higher. Is there any way to raise it? Unfortunately, you have a small degree of control over your RMR, since it is determined primarily by your body size. The larger you are, the higher your RMR. But you can increase your RMR a little if you add muscle mass to your body. This is one reason why some weight-management experts advocate resistance exercise such as weight lifting. Each pound of muscle you add will increase your RMR. It's not easy to add muscle mass, however. Sure, if you become a bodybuilder and devote hours each day to weight lifting, you can add a lot of muscle mass. But most of us won't be able to add enough muscle mass with weight lifting to increase our RMR very much. Nonetheless, a lot of successful weight-loss maintainers do engage in some resistance exercise.

You may have also heard that RMR increases after exercise. This is true, but the increase usually occurs only after very vigorous physical activity performed for a long period of time. Again, for most of you, this will not be an important factor in your total energy expenditure.

> **MYTH: LEAN PEOPLE HAVE A HIGHER METABOLISM THAN OVERWEIGHT PEOPLE**
>
> In fact, the opposite is true. Heavier people have a higher metabolism than lighter people. When you gain weight, your metabolism goes up, and when you lose weight, your metabolism goes down.

You may have also seen advertisements for products that "boost" your metabolism. It will come as no surprise that none of these products have

> **AMAZING FACT**
>
> For every pound of weight you lose, your resting metabolism goes down by about 8 calories a day.

any research behind them to prove that they work for long-term weight loss. They sound too good to be true, and they probably are.

2. The Thermic Effect of Food (TEF)

TEF is the rise in heat production and body temperature that occurs after you eat. This is the amount of energy your body burns in order to convert the energy contained in food into forms of energy that the body uses for essential functions. The "burning" is why you sometimes feel warm after eating a large meal.

TEF typically represents less than 10 percent of the total food energy you consume. So, if you eat 2,000 calories in a day, fewer than 200 are given off as heat in the thermic effect of food. The thermic effect is greatest for dietary protein and least for fat. Thus, TEF will be a little lower if you are consuming a very high-fat diet as compared to a lower-fat diet. This is another good reason to avoid eating a very high-fat diet.

Since the thermic effect is a relatively small component of total daily energy expenditure and you are not able to control it, it is not an important part of the Step Diet. But it will be reduced slightly if you reduce your energy intake to lose weight.

3. Energy Expended in Physical Activity

Although you have very little ability to increase your RMR or TEF, you have almost total control over the energy you expend through physical activity. Here is where you have the best opportunity to increase your total energy expenditure.

AMAZING FACT

Most overweight people burn less than 20 percent of their total daily calories during physical activity.

When you engage in physical activity, you burn more fuel to provide your muscles with the extra energy needed for the activity. All muscular work burns energy. When you stand, you burn more energy than when you sit—it takes muscular work to stand and maintain your balance. You burn more sitting than lying down, and so forth. Of course, there are much bigger increases above resting energy expenditure in the amount of energy it takes to walk, run, ride a bicycle, swim, play tennis, or lift a significant amount of weight. This is because you use more muscles more intensively in these activities. The more muscles you use, the more energy you burn, and of course, the more intensively you use these muscles, the more energy you burn in a given amount of time.

So, unlike your resting metabolism, which varies between people of similar size due to genetic variation, it takes the same amount of energy for two similar-sized people to walk a mile. Finally, you can do something to improve your weight!

The energy burned in physical activities in which you move your body over some distance (such as walking, running, cycling, swimming, or playing tennis, soccer, or golf) is related to your body weight. It takes more energy to move a larger weight than a smaller one. Of course, you also burn energy in other kinds of activities in which you don't move your whole body (pulling weeds in the garden, scrubbing floors, lifting weights, etc.). With the exception of weight training, these activities of daily living don't burn nearly as much energy as moving your whole body—and they are very difficult to monitor. You might consider such activities as bonus energy expenditure that will help accelerate your weight loss and make it easier to maintain your weight.

How Energy Is Stored in the Body

Energy can be stored in the body in the form of protein, carbohydrates, and fat.

1. Protein is stored largely in muscle tissue and is not available for energy expenditure except during starvation.

2. The body can store only about one day's supply of carbohydrate. Carbohydrates are stored in the form of glycogen in muscle and in the liver, and they circulate in the form of glucose in the blood. (Glycogen and glucose are great sources of fuel for the body's metabolism, but there is not much around.)

3. The body has an unlimited ability to store fat in adipose tissue (body fat). Fat is also a great source of fuel for the body, and there is plenty of it around.

Because protein stores are not very changeable, and because so few carbohydrates are stored in the body, when you gain or lose weight, most of that weight—about 70 to 80 percent—is body fat. The other 20 percent is mostly protein.

It takes about 3,500 calories of negative energy balance to lose 1 pound of body weight. If you want to lose 10 pounds, you need to create a total negative energy balance of 35,000 calories. We have told you that a weight loss rate of 1 to 2 pounds per week is best. So, let's say you wante to lose 1 pound in a week. You would need to burn 500 calories more than you eat for each day over seven days. To lose 2 pounds a week, the upper end of recommended safe weight loss, you would need to burn 1,000 calories more per day than you eat.

Develop Your Energy Balance Skills

By now you should understand the main components of energy balance, but the key is knowing how to change your behavior to achieve the state of energy balance that you want. Think of managing your energy balance just as you manage your finances. To manage your finances, you need some basic knowledge about the value of money and how much things cost. To manage your energy balance, you need to know the value of food and physical activity and how one relates to the other. Just as you decide whether you can afford that new pair of boots this month, you need to consider whether you can afford a food choice, given your level of energy expenditure. Since your amount of physical activity is the part of energy expenditure you have most control over, whether you can afford a particular food choice may relate to how many steps you have accumulated.

It is important to realize that in the short term you can control much more energy on the intake side than on the expenditure side of the energy balance equation. You have control over everything you eat but over only a portion (10–50 percent) of your expenditure—this is energy expended in physical activity. As shown in the following table, there is no contest between your ability to modify your energy intake and your ability to modify your physical activity. You can take in a lot of energy in a very short period of time! To burn this amount of energy will take much longer. It works the same in producing negative energy balance. You can easily eat 560 fewer calories on any given day, but it takes a long time to burn 560 calories. This is why so many people who give weight-loss advice focus primarily on the intake side—you can get results quickly. The problem is, these results are short-lived. Increasing physical activity does not give the immediate results, but it is critical in the long term.

ENERGY INTAKE VERSUS ENERGY EXPENDITURE			
Activity	Calories Gained or Lost	Duration	Efficiency (Calories per Minute)
Eat a Big Mac	Gained 560 calories	3 minutes	Gained 187 calories per minute
Exercise at 70 percent of maximum	Burned 560 calories	60 minutes	Burned about 9 calories per minute
Exercise at 40 percent of maximum	Burned 560 calories	90 minutes	Burned about 6 calories per minute

You have to prioritize managing your energy balance just as you must prioritize managing your finances. You must devote enough time to make sure it is done right. If you are ignoring your finances, you're setting the stage for a bad outcome. If you ignore your weight management, it is likely that bad things will happen there as well. It is easier to manage your finances once you get them in "good shape." And it is certainly easier to manage your weight once you get it into good shape. We have shown you a simple way to manage the energy through your body—using the MegaSteps Energy Balance method.

Your Body Helps Maintain Energy Balance

The average adult eats between 1,500 and 3,000 calories each day, depending on body size and amount of physical activity. This amounts to a yearly intake of between 500,000 and 1,000,000 calories. In order to maintain stable body weight over the course of a year, the same amount of energy must be expended.

As we discussed, gaining a pound of body fat represents an excess of energy intake over expenditure of 3,500 calories. This means that over the course of a year, if you eat only 10 calories a day more than you burn—one LifeSaver!—you will gain a pound of body weight. If your body's biological mechanism for balancing energy intake and expenditure unconsciously were in error by just 1 percent (that is, you consistently eat 1 percent more than you burn), there would be a positive energy imbalance of between 15 and 30 calories a day that would result in a weight gain of 1^1/$_2$ to 3 pounds of body fat per year. So don't get down on yourself for having bad genes—even if you are gaining weight, your body does a pretty good job of helping you match intake with expenditure. You would probably consider a 1 percent error rate (99 percent reliability) pretty good for a mechanical device you use every day, such as an automobile, a refrigerator, or your home computer.

The good news is that our bodies are better at automatically balancing energy intake and expenditure than we realize—in other words, everyone has some natural capacity to manage body weight. The bad news is that in the environment we live in, this unconscious mechanism is no longer enough to keep body weight stable at a healthy level, and those small imbalances (10, 15, 20 calories a day) accumulate over the years. Before you know it, you are tipping the scales at 10 to 20 pounds more than a healthy weight.

Achieving energy balance in today's world requires using our brains—in effect, we must go from relying on instinct to balance food intake and energy expenditure to using our intellect to overcome the forces in the environment that constantly push us to eat too much and move too little. We showed you how to do this to lose weight, by making small changes to eat a little less and move a little more. You also need to use your brain to help with keeping your weight off.

CHAPTER 8

Do It Again

If you succeeded in losing weight and keeping it off the first time around, and you want to lose more weight, you may be ready for another cycle of weight loss and maintenance. But before you begin on a second (or third) twelve-week weight-loss cycle, you have to make sure you have a solid plan. You have to ask yourself whether you can sustain more behavior changes. Sure, you can lose more weight—but will you be able to keep this additional weight off? How difficult is it for you to keep off the weight you lost the first time around? If you are struggling to keep this weight off, it will be even harder to keep more weight off. Remember, to change your weight, you have to change your genes, your behavior, or your environment. You already know that you can't change your genes, but you may be able to change your behavior or your environment. Are you ready and willing to make more changes in order to lose and keep off more weight?

Luckily, the overall strategy for losing more weight is the same as for losing weight during the initial twelve-week phase—eating a little less and moving a little more. But your expectations need to change—after all, you've already increased your steps for your first weight loss, and now you'll have to increase your step count even more if you want to maintain a greater weight loss. Can you keep your total energy expenditure (your BodySteps plus your LifeSteps) constant during weight loss to counter your drop in metabolism? This may mean increasing your steps by another 500 LifeSteps per day over the next twelve weeks (a total of 6,000 more steps per day). Think about how this can happen.

> **PLAN FOR THE ENDGAME, NOT THE TEMPORARY SOLUTION**
>
> Make sure you are ready for another twelve-week weight-loss period. If you can't make additional changes in your lifestyle, you can't keep off more weight.

If you cannot increase your steps this much, you may not be able to totally compensate for any further drop in your metabolic rate without further reducing your food intake. This means that your weight loss may not be as great during additional cycles of weight loss, and you will need to adjust your expectations accordingly.

If time is the reason you cannot increase your steps, you can consider more intense forms of activity (such as jogging or cycling) that burn more energy (MegaSteps) per minute than walking. This way, you can get more total energy expenditure for the same amount of time. Just make sure that you choose an activity that you enjoy and can envision doing permanently.

Even if you cannot increase your physical activity any more, you may still be able to lose a significant amount of weight by reducing your energy intake by 25 percent. Just keep in mind that you must be prepared to

Success Story 12

Brittany's Smart Choice

Brittany lost 20 pounds during her first twelve-week weight-loss period—10 pounds less than her weight-loss goal. After weight loss, she worked hard to find her personal energy balance point. She struggled to get her LifeSteps consistently above 10,000 per day, and she had to pay attention to portion sizes and occasionally use the 75 percent rule. After six weeks, she was confident that she could maintain her weight loss using the Step Diet. She then decided to go through another twelve-week period to lose the additional 10 pounds. However, after reading Chapters 6 and 7, she decided that she wasn't sure she could make the further lifestyle changes she would have to make to lose more weight. She was confident she could keep the 20 pounds off but not confident she could do more. Brittany decided that she could be satisfied both with her new weight and with the lifestyle that maintained it.

permanently eat less food in order to maintain your weight loss. That's because your metabolic rate will drop further with additional weight loss. If you cannot compensate for this lowered metabolism by walking more, you will have to maintain a reduced food intake to lose weight. If you rely primarily on eating less to lose weight this time around, you will likely have to rely on it more to keep the weight off as well. The major problem with this tactic is excessive hunger. If hunger becomes a problem when you are trying to maintain your second (or third) weight loss, you can use some of the tips in Appendix A to increase the quality

NEW CYCLE, DIFFERENT EXPECTATIONS

Losing weight during a new weight-loss cycle can be more challenging than the first cycle. Here are some things to keep in mind so you don't get frustrated—or overdo it:

- Remember the basic rules of energy balance: If calorie intake increases, exercise must increase; if exercise decreases, calorie intake must decrease.

- If you don't have time to devote to more walking, try a more strenuous exercise (running, cycling, etc.) that burns more calories per minute.

- Try replacing some current foods with fat-free versions, if possible—for example, switch from ice cream to frozen yogurt, or use ground turkey instead of ground beef when making spaghetti sauce or taco filling.

of your diet. Reducing the energy density of your diet, for example, will allow you to eat a greater total weight of food while getting less energy.

Your second (or third) weight-loss cycle should not be longer than twelve weeks. While you might be tempted to extend the cycle, it will not help in the long term. You will do better if you work hard at losing weight for a defined period of time, then stop losing and concentrate on keeping it off.

You can also consider whether you can change your environment to make it easier to lose more weight. Can you put yourself in a position where you get some physical activity every day without having to think about it? Can you, for example, change the way you go to work? Can you walk part of the way or ride your bike? Can you join a tennis or golf league or commit to some other activity that ensures you get some additional physical activity on a regular basis?

Can you change your food environment? Can you permanently reduce the number of times you eat out during the week? Can you make permanent changes in the type of diet you eat? You might find that a change in your environment helps you make the additional behavior changes you need to lose more weight and keep it off.

Success Story 13

Finding the Balance Point

Charles lost 23 pounds in his first twelve-week weight loss period. With the feedback from his step counter, Charles found that he could get his daily LifeSteps to 12,000 and, on many days, even higher. After weight loss, he started playing tennis twice a week and golf every other weekend. He even went jogging every now and then. This increased his LifeStep total even more. He didn't have to use the 75 percent rule to keep his weight off; he just watched his portions and tried to eat only when he was hungry. He found it surprisingly easy to maintain his weight loss and decided to try another twelve-week weight-loss period. On his second weight-loss try, Charles lost another 15 pounds. He had to work a little harder to keep this weight off, but because he had been able to increase his physical activity so much, he was able to keep off 12 of these additional 15 pounds. Charles reached a weight and lifestyle that he could live with forever.

Success Story 14
Don't Give Up or Give In

JoAnn had a BMI of 45 and wanted to lose over 100 pounds. She was seriously considering gastric bypass surgery for weight loss, but her husband convinced her to try the Step Diet. Initially she was not very happy about having to stop losing weight after twelve weeks and about aiming for only 1 to 2 pounds of weight loss per week—but she tried it. She lost 30 pounds during her first weight-loss period—a little more than 2 pounds per week. She kept it off easily by watching portions and passive overeating and getting in a little more walking. Still, she could only get her LifeSteps up to about 8,000 per day. After keeping her weight off for six weeks, she tried another period of weight loss. This time she lost 24 pounds. Again, she found it fairly easy to keep the weight off, this time by using the MegaSteps Energy Balance methods. Now she was getting over 10,000 LifeSteps per day. After another three months, she tried a third period of weight loss and lost another 10 pounds, which she found she could keep off. JoAnn had lost 64 pounds. This was short of her goal, but she felt so good, she decided against the surgery. She hopes to try a fourth period of weight loss sometime next year. She is optimistic that eventually she will reach her goal.

How Long Should You Wait between Weight-Loss Cycles?

Some of you, especially those with large amounts of weight to lose, may be eager to start another weight-loss cycle soon after your first one. Is this a good idea? There is no right answer for everyone. Before you consider doing so, you must be sure that you can keep off the weight lost during the first cycle. A good rule of thumb is that you should maintain your weight loss for at least four weeks before trying to lose more weight. If you are finding it difficult to achieve your personal energy balance point, you may want to wait even longer before beginning a second weight-loss cycle—possibly a year or more. It all depends on your comfort zone; if you're not totally comfortable with maintaining your first weight loss, chances are you won't maintain a greater weight loss.

SUCCESS TIP

Maintain your weight loss for at least four weeks before trying to lose more weight.

Getting Started

Additional cycles of the Step Diet begin with setting new weight-management goals. Start with Stage 1 of the Step Diet, just as you did before, with seven days of recording your food intake and steps per day. Then move directly to Stage 3. Reread Chapter 4 to make sure you are clear on your weight-management goals. Once you've set your target, start by using the 75 percent strategy (Stage 4) and increasing your steps, if possible. Stages 5 and 6 are just as important this time as before—there's no point in losing weight if you cannot keep it off. Your approach to maintenance after the second or third round of weight loss should be the same as before, too—stabilizing your weight by burning more energy by raising daily LifeSteps to the highest maintainable level, adjusting

**WEIGHT IN
THE BALANCE**

Your personal energy balance point
will clearly change with more weight
loss.

food intake with portion control, and managing hunger with the use of free foods. Also, keep adhering to the principles of Stage 5, including weighing yourself regularly. In addition, you should reread Chapter 7 and Appendix A to consider additional small changes you can make to take some of the strain out of maintaining your personal energy balance point.

There's technically no limit to how many weight-loss cycles you can go through—as long as you can maintain your last weight loss before trying for more. Successful weight loss and maintenance are all about consistency. And you may find, over time, that consistency depends not just on rigorous attention to your eating and exercise behavior, but on the fact that your weight-management plan has become almost an automatic part of your life. After all, you don't have to work very hard to wash your face or brush your teeth every day, do you?

CHAPTER 9

A New You

The Step Diet is much more than just a twelve-week weight-loss program. It's really a new lease on life—a life of improved control over your eating patterns and activity that can have major positive benefits on your health and even your outlook on life. Maintaining this control, however, can seem like a lot of work—unless you can make it part of the normal flow of your day. This becomes more critical with the more weight you have lost. Losing 50 pounds is fundamentally different from losing 5 pounds just to fit into your favorite dress or sport jacket. You might be able to lose 5 pounds by making very minor changes to your life and possibly without anyone else even knowing that you are attempting weight loss. Losing and maintaining much more weight loss will require the kinds of behavior change that will be noticed by those around you. You will have transformed your lifestyle. Because of these changes, you will appear to yourself and others as a different person—the New You.

Creating a New Identity

For many of you, especially those who have lost a lot of weight, lasting success in weight management will come from creating a new identity for yourself—one in which the behaviors that enable you to maintain a healthy weight take on a broader meaning for you than weight control. You can find connections between these key behaviors and other aspects of your life that are important to you. You are enhancing your emotional and spiritual self in addition to your mental and physical self. You can reach a state where you need these behaviors to maintain a life balance that goes far beyond weight control.

One of the best ways to succeed over the long term with the Step Diet is to reach a state in which your new behaviors become so folded into your life that they require no special attention. Then you will not be on a "program" or permanent diet; you will be living a new lifestyle, one in which eating less and moving more are not chores or temporary rituals. Even if the new behaviors are small changes from what you did before, they are still different—and as such, they can be difficult to maintain. Managing to find connections between these new behaviors and other important aspects of your life will help you immeasurably.

After conducting extensive interviews with people who have succeeded in long-term weight management, we have found that the degree to which people recompose their lives as fit and healthy individuals is a powerful indicator of success. Indeed, the most successful individuals had found a balance among four life factors: physical, emotional, mental, and spiritual.

The New You Must Use Both Sides of Your Brain

Losing weight by finding a balance between energy intake and expenditure is a very analytical process. It requires that you use your left brain to keep track of a seemingly endless stream of numbers—on the bathroom scale, on your step counter, on the nutrition labels of the food you eat. Though it is certainly possible to use this information alone to achieve success over the long haul, isn't there more to life? Who wants to worry constantly about keeping track of their eating and physical activity in order to maintain a healthy body weight? You want your life to be fulfilling and

> **GO WITH THE FLOW**
>
> Barbara had her normal share of stress as a harried New Yorker—at home and on the job. She coped by eating; she said it made her happy. After losing 100 pounds, Barbara found a new place to make herself happy: the pool at her new gym. After a hard day at work, she "washes off" her stress by walking in the pool (that's right, walking—it's even lower impact when you do it underwater). The gym also provides a reflective interlude after work before she goes home to her three kids.

enjoyable on many levels. This means finding connections between the many different components of your life that help define who you are. Many people want to find stronger connections to others and their community, and these tasks require use of your right brain.

The Physical Factor

Exercise and the creative integration of movement into daily life, as well as behaviors related to eating, are what we think of as the physical factor. Nearly every person who succeeds in long-term weight management acknowledges that physical activity is at the core of their success—and is also critically important to their spiritual and emotional well-being. Many of them use their exercise time to reflect and meditate. Some even use it for prayer. Most important, they seem to place a higher meaning on physical activity in their lives than they had before. They found a link between the act of performing physical activity and the fulfillment of other important needs, whether they were spiritual, emotional, or mental. No longer were they doing physical activity simply for the purpose of burning energy and managing body weight. Being active became an identifying feature of who they are.

The Emotional Factor

Having contact and shared commitments with other people is not just important for preventing loneliness, it is key for externalizing emotions. Without these connections, negative feelings about yourself or your situation turn inward, fueling self-destructive behavior, such as eating to feel good or becoming lethargic and inactive. If you lose significant amounts of weight, you should examine whether your previous emotional support systems actually support your new lifestyle. Some successful weight-loss maintainers have sought out social groups that revolve around physical activity rather than eating. It is important that you make healthy emotional connections. Some people find healthy connections in an active social life, others in support systems like church organizations or gyms. Job satisfaction, hobbies, and other creative endeavors are all crucial sources of emotional strength. Find those sources of strength that reinforce the new lifestyle you have chosen. And let's not forget that our pets can provide significant emotional support—and even practical help. What can motivate a walk more than a dog begging to go out?

The Mental Factor

Congratulations! You've set new goals, expanded your self-confidence, and believed in your ultimate success. Think of a time that you've made a list of things to do, no matter what they were. Remember how you felt when you checked off the last thing on the list? You felt a sense of accomplishment, and you felt good. And you were ready to make a new list!

Successful weight-loss maintainers are constantly challenging themselves to set new goals. They are not afraid to experiment. It is unlikely that you will build the self-confidence needed to gain control over the behaviors that promote weight gain unless you challenge yourself to change and constantly explore new ways to create a lifestyle that is consonant with fitness and health—but is still uniquely you. The ability to build structure into life is also a common characteristic of successful individuals. The structuring of daily or weekly living makes sticking to new behaviors easier. For example, if you get into the habit of eating only 75 percent of the food on your plate instead of everything, you will dramatically improve your chances of maintaining a healthy weight.

The mental factor and the physical factor are commonly intertwined, as people often report that physical activity clears their mind and helps them focus not only on their goals but also on bringing other aspects of their life into balance. The next time you face a challenging mental task, take a walk while you work through it.

The Spiritual Factor

For some people, spirituality is a belief in a higher power. This belief system can provide strong support as people progress through the transformational process of losing weight. Spirituality can also be a channel for stress release, whether or not formal religion is involved. It can take the shape of meditation or yoga, activities that allow you to temporarily escape from your hectic day-to-day life. The inner calm that comes from any kind of spiritual activity reenergizes you while also, sometimes, providing a beneficial structure to daily or weekly life.

Learn to find the links between the healthy behaviors you want to maintain and other important aspects of your life. Make the changes in your daily life part of who you are. A journey of a thousand miles, said Lao-tzu, begins with a single step. On your journey, you have learned to step your way to lower weight and improved health.

Change Your Environment

You already know that the environment we live in pushes many of us to overeat and to be physically inactive. We have found that

Success Story 15
Passing the Bar

As a young professor in Boston, Timothy frequently went to pubs, and drinking and eating with friends was an integral part of his identity. At 6 feet tall, he topped 270 pounds before he realized, with the help of a doctor, that he needed to lose weight. Timothy lost 90 pounds, but he was having trouble keeping it off. One thing was certain: He could not go back to his old social life. Timothy decided to take a research year in San Diego, where he had some family. In the sunshine of his new environment, he made walking a big part of his daily routine.

When he moved back to Boston ten months later, he enjoyed the company of his old friends away from the pubs, and he looked for new friends as walking partners. Timothy now walks not only to maintain his weight but also to sustain his newfound mental and emotional strength. At 180 pounds, he is a different person from the man who weighed 270 pounds.

many of our successful weight-loss maintainers have learned to create a "mini" healthy environment for themselves within their larger external environment. Some have changed their hobbies or even their careers to incorporate healthy eating and active living. Some have taken up cooking or gardening. Some have gone back to school to learn about nutrition, and a few have actually become dietitians. Others have taken up active hobbies such as mountain biking, canoeing, or even mountain climbing. Some have become physical activity teachers in schools.

You don't have to change careers or even change hobbies to maintain your weight loss. You do have to realize that you are not "cured." You will always have to be concerned about not gaining your weight back. People in the National Weight Control Registry, even those who have maintained their weight loss for thirty or forty years, are still concerned about gaining their weight back. They feel confident in their ability to keep it off, but they do think about it. The more you can change your personal environment to one that supports healthier lifestyle choices, the easier it will be for you to keep your weight off. Look around your community, talk with others who live a similar lifestyle, and experiment with ways to create your own healthy "mini" environment.

The Step Diet at Your Workplace

Many of you spend a lot of time at work. The workplace is an environment that is very conducive to implementing the Step Diet. Forming walking groups to get your steps in and help each other with the 75 percent rule in your company cafeteria or in nearby restaurants is a simple, inexpensive way to lose weight with your co-workers. Some companies post signs giving the number of steps it takes to get from one part of the work site to another or to local coffeeshops or restaurants. Often, employers will help by providing incentives for employees who succeed in losing weight and keeping it off with the Step Diet.

The Step Diet for Life

The small changes we advocate in the Step Diet are changes that can improve health and the quality of life for you and your family. This is not just a way to lose weight and keep it off, nor a way to prevent weight gain. It is a better way to live. Help your family members adopt healthier eating and physical activity patterns that will benefit them throughout their lives. Teach your children and grandchildren the importance of staying physically active, whether by walking, playing sports, or engaging in less structured activities in the neighborhood and throughout the community. Teach them to pay attention to how much they are eating at meals, and teach them about appropriate portion sizes. Expose them to a variety of healthy food choices and help them discover how to improve their eating habits. If we all do this, we will begin raising a generation of healthy children, free from the problems of overweight. Set a good example. (Despite what we tell our children, they do persist in imitating us.)

And then congratulate yourself.

You've successfully integrated the principles of the Step Diet into your life. You've taken stock of your weight situation, taken action to manage it, and forged a permanent new identity for yourself as an active, health-conscious person. If you have reached this point, we're sure you'll continue to follow in the footsteps of others who have found new well-being and self-esteem with the Step Diet. Just keep putting one foot in front of the other. . . .

Happy walking!

Energy Awareness

You don't count calories on the Step Diet. You just make sure that the MegaSteps in the foods you eat are less than (or equal to) your daily MegaSteps of energy expenditure. One way to do this is to eat smarter, and to stop the passive overeating that fuels much of our weight gain. Now that you have lost weight by eating a little less and have achieved a balance between MegaSteps in and MegaSteps out, you might want to think about making better food choices, which may in turn reduce the total MegaSteps you consume. However, remember to make only those that you can live with forever. There's no point in making temporary changes that will give temporary results.

This section is filled with tips for improving the quality of your diet. Browse through it and see which ones are useful for you. Look for small changes that can easily be incorporated into your daily life. Remember that these tips are just suggestions—none of them is necessary for long-term weight management. But some of them may make it much easier.

Breakfast Smarts

• Make sure you eat breakfast every single day. People who eat breakfast eat fewer total calories during the day.

• Cereal, fruit, and pancakes are good breakfast choices.

• Choose the high-fiber, low-sugar types of cereals.

• Leave the butter off pancakes, waffles, or French toast and save 90 calories.

• Waffles: Don't eat one square and save 60 calories.

• French toast: If you eat one and a half slices of bread instead of two, you'll save 40 calories.

• Scrambled eggs: Make with one whole egg and one egg white instead of two whole eggs to save 80 calories.

Lunch Smarts

Sandwiches are good lunch choices. Here are some tips:

• Leave off one slice of lunch meat and save 65 calories.

• Have an open-faced sandwich and save 90 calories.

• Leave off the mayo and save 100 calories.

When eating lunch at a fast-food restaurant:

- Take out one hamburger patty in the double hamburger and save 200 calories, or don't eat one bun and save 60 calories.

- Order the small hamburger instead of the double hamburger and save 150 calories.

- Order the four-piece chicken nuggets instead of the six-piece and save 100 calories.

- Eat ten fewer french fries or, even better, order the small french fries instead of the medium and save 240 calories.

When ordering entrée salads (we're using examples from Applebee's menu), here's how to make sure "only a salad" doesn't take up more than half your daily calories:

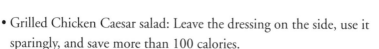

SUCCESS TIP

Did you know that a taco salad with dressing has more than twice the calories of a chicken burrito?

- Asian Chicken or Blackened Chicken salad: Choose the "regular" instead of the "large" size and save more than 250 calories.

- Grilled Chicken Caesar salad: Leave the dressing on the side, use it sparingly, and save more than 100 calories.

- Chinese Chicken salad: Leave off the chow mein noodles and save 120 calories.

- Taco salad: Don't eat the shell and save yourself 180 calories.

- Cobb salad: Eat half of the blue cheese and half of the crumbled bacon and save more than 200 calories.

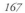

Learn to Manage Salad Bars

Now, let's look at how you can use portion control to better manage a salad bar.

You get a savings of 359 calories in just one meal! As you can see, we upped or kept the portion size on the free foods (marked with asterisks) and decreased the portion size on the higher-calorie foods. This way, you still feel like you are eating a large amount of food, but you're not getting the extra calories.

Food	TYPICAL SALAD BAR		PORTION CONTROL SALAD BAR	
	Amount	**Calories**	**Amount**	**Calories**
LETTUCE*	1 1/2 cups	15	2 cups	20
CARROTS*	1/4 cup	12	1/2 cup	25
CUCUMBERS*	1/2 cup slices	5	1 cup slices	10
MUSHROOMS*	1/2 cup slices	20	1/2 cup slices	20
TOMATOES*	1/2 cup slices	10	1/2 cup slices	10
ANTIPASTO SALAD	1/2 cup	70	1/4 cup	35
BEAN SALAD	1/2 cup	110	1/4 cup	55
CARROT AND RAISIN SALAD	1/2 cup	65	1/4 cup	33
POTATO SALAD	1/2 cup	160	1/4 cup	80
BACON BITS	2 tablespoons	60	1 tablespoon	30
CHOW MEIN NOODLES	1/2 cup	120	1/4 cup	60
RANCH DRESSING	3 tablespoons	270	2 tablespoons	180
TOTAL CALORIES		**952**		**593**

Dinner Smarts

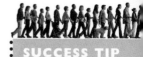

SUCCESS TIP

Most of us consume the majority of our calories in the evening, making it even more important to watch portion sizes at night. Check out these simple tips for making sure you don't overdo it.

Did you know that the average salad dressing ladle at a salad bar contains 3 tablespoons? If you chose a regular ranch dressing, this would deliver 270 extra calories to an otherwise healthy meal. Use 1 tablespoon and save 180 calories!

• Chicken: Cut the meat off the bone and then eat a reasonable portion. The leftover chicken makes a great sandwich, casserole, or stir-fry. If you take the skin off the chicken before cooking it, you can save more than 100 calories. If you take the skin off after cooking, you will save 50 calories.

• Beef: Choose the leaner cuts of beef to save additional calories and consume less saturated fat. This includes extra-lean hamburger meat, filet mignon, and flank steak. Cutting off the visible fat from your meat can also reduce calories and fat intake. For instance, if you trim the fat off a round steak before eating it, you will save more than 50 calories.

• Pasta dishes: Consider the toppings on your pasta as well. If you are eating spaghetti with meatballs, eat only half the meatballs. Certain types of pasta sauces can also add calories and fat. As an example, fettuccine Alfredo has 910 calories compared with the same serving of spaghetti with marinara sauce, which has only 540 calories.

• Potatoes: Reduce the amount of butter, margarine, or sour cream. Even better, try fat-free sour cream or top with fat-free ranch dressing or salsa and save up to 100 calories.

• Mashed potatoes: Try using skim milk or evaporated skim milk in your mashed potato recipe and reduce your calories by 80.

TAKE ACTION AGAINST PASSIVE OVEREATING

We all bite off more than we should chew once in a while. Here are some more tips on how to cut down on calories when you're eating out:

- Split your entrée with someone else at the table.

- Consider ordering an appetizer as a main course.

- Avoid "pre-eating"—that is, indulging in the breadbasket or other freebies on the table while you wait for your main meal.

• Rice: Decrease the amount of butter or margarine you add and save up to 100 calories.

• Vegetables: Here is where you can load up on those free foods. We suggest that you steam your vegetables to retain flavor and vitamin content. Just watch how much butter, margarine, or salad dressing you use and save up to 100 calories.

Smart Drinks

Most people do not include the beverages they drink in the equation when thinking about their caloric intake—but these can add up. Check this out:

• Soda, 12 ounces = 150 calories

• Coffee, 2 cups with cream = 90 calories

• Starbucks Mocha Frappuccino, grande = 320 calories

• Orange juice, 8 ounces = 115 calories

Success Story 16

Cutting Calories During Cocktail Hour

Jane was always so hungry and stressed when she got home from work that she would have a couple of glasses of wine and some cheese and crackers before dinner every night. The wine really helped her to relax, but Jane was taking in a lot of calories before she even sat down to the dinner table. So she changed her predinner menu. Now she eats a light snack at 4:00 P.M., then has one glass of wine when she comes home. This way, she still gets to relax, but she's not hungry enough to eat a big snack before dinner.

- Odwalla "C" Monster, 8 ounces = 300 calories

- Gatorade, 12 ounces = 90 calories

- Beer, 12 ounces = 140 calories

- Wine, 6 ounces = 125 calories

- Strawberry daiquiri, 12 ounces = 220 calories

To reduce the calories you consume in beverages, try these tips:

- Choose water or a noncaloric beverage such as diet soda, club soda, iced tea, or a powdered, noncaloric sweetened beverage.

- Limit fruit juices and sports drinks to 4 to 6 ounces per day. You can mix the juice with extra water or seltzer to dilute the calories.

• Limit alcohol to one drink per day. Dilute your alcohol with club soda or diet soda (wine spritzer or gin and tonic, heavy on the tonic).

Tricks of the Trade

• Eat slowly. It takes a while before our brain registers that we are full. Often, if you wait a few minutes before going for seconds, you'll find you don't want them.

• Use smaller bowls and plates. This can give you the perception that your plate is full.

• Leave serving bowls in the kitchen. Don't put extra food on the table—it's too tempting to eat more food when it's right in front of you.

• Keep food out of sight at home and work. Don't keep candy or nuts on the kitchen counter or on your desk. Put them in your pantry or in a cabinet where you can't see them. The sight of food is a strong stimulus to eat more.

• Don't use food as a reward. If you are feeling stressed or have had a hard day, reward yourself with a hot bath, a massage, or a walk. You will reduce the stress without the calories.

ARE MEAL REPLACEMENTS USEFUL?

Meal replacements, usually in liquid form, are a way of ensuring portion control at meals. There's nothing wrong with them, they come in many flavors, and research has shown that they can be useful in managing calorie intake and weight. In fact, recent results from researchers at Harvard and UCLA suggest meal replacements may be helpful in long-term maintenance of weight loss. In times of stress, when you need more structure in your eating, meal replacements may be a convenient and good-tasting alternative. Other people may want to use them on a regular basis to replace meals. It's up to you.

Success Story 17

Adding "Action!" to Movie Night

Marcia's family's tradition on Sundays was to meet for an early dinner and then watch a movie. They decided to offer more low-fat, low-calorie choices to their weekly dinner, and then go for a walk after dinner and before the movie. They even started a family competition around who can accumulate the greatest number of steps!

• Plan family and social gatherings around physical activity rather than food. Plan to meet friends for a hike, bike ride, or bowling.

Tips to Decrease Fats and Sweets

Since you reduce your intake by 9 calories for each gram of fat you take out of your diet and 4 calories for each gram of sugar, you may want to try these tips to eliminate some fats and sweets.

• Limit dressing on salads to 1 tablespoon or switch to low-fat or fat-free dressing.

• Use just a little less butter, margarine, and mayonnaise.

• Use less gravy and sauces that add fat to other foods.

• Use less sour cream and cream cheese or use the low-fat or fat-free versions.

• For a snack, have a piece of fruit, a small box of raisins, some pretzels, or a light yogurt in place of candy or chips.

• Limit your intake of doughnuts, sweet rolls, high-fat muffins, and croissants. It is easy to overeat these foods. Substitute whole-grain cereals, breads, waffles, bagels, or English muffins.

• In place of cookies, cakes, or other dessert pastries, have a few graham crackers, gingersnaps, or animal crackers. Other good substitutes are juice-packed canned fruit, applesauce, frozen fruit bars, or low-calorie fudge bars.

Tips to Increase Fruits and Vegetables

Research suggests that a diet high in fruits and vegetables—good sources of fiber, vitamins, and minerals—can help prevent many chronic diseases, such as cancer and heart disease. And it's very hard to overeat fruits and vegetables!

• Eat a minimum of five servings of fruits and vegetables each day. Most vegetables are considered "free" foods; fruits and vegetables also have the added benefit of being very low density foods. Eating several servings each day will take the edge off your appetite and help you control your portion sizes of higher-calorie foods.

• Keep small cans of 100 percent fruit juice at work to have as a snack.

• Keep fresh fruits visible in the refrigerator and on the countertop.

• Use fresh, canned, or dried fruit as toppings for cereal, pancakes, waffles, and French toast. Thawed frozen berries or raisins make easy toppers.

• Add thawed frozen berries to plain or vanilla yogurt.

• Have 6 ounces of 100 percent fruit juice with breakfast. Mix 100 percent fruit juices with sparkling water or club soda as an after-dinner drink or snack.

• Blend fresh or frozen fruits with low-fat milk or yogurt to make a fruit smoothie.

• Pack fresh, canned, or dried fruit for snacks. Dried fruits such as raisins, prunes, apricots, apple slices, and cranberries are excellent choices.

• Put raisins, mandarin oranges, grapes, or apple chunks into salads.

• At work, keep small cans of water-packed fruit on hand.

• Freeze fresh bananas, grapes, or strawberries and serve partially thawed for a dessert.

• Look for fresh fruits in salad bars, or start with a fresh fruit cup when eating out.

• Have a small can of vegetable juice as a snack.

• Buy prepackaged raw vegetables and use for a snack with a low-fat dip.

• Make an egg-white omelet with tomatoes, mushrooms, onions, green peppers, and other raw or canned vegetables.

• Include a mixed green salad or vegetable soup with your lunch or dinner.

• Keep frozen vegetables on hand and microwave them for an easy side dish at lunch or dinner.

• Add extra vegetables to your frozen meals, soups, or other ready-made packaged or canned items. Canned and frozen vegetables are easy to use.

• Once a week, make a batch of soup that includes lots of vegetables.

• Order sandwiches or wraps that include several vegetables, such as lettuce, tomatoes, sprouts, green pepper, cucumber, and other raw vegetables.

• Make your own pizza with lots of vegetable toppings.

• Double the amount of vegetables you eat at dinner.

Tips to Increase Fiber

Plant foods contain two different types of fiber categorized by how
soluble they are in water. Most plant foods contain both types of
fiber, but they vary in the amounts of each. Insoluble fibers, as the
name suggests, are not soluble in water and they help to create a soft
bulk and hasten the passage of waste products through the intestine.
The best food sources of insoluble fiber are wheat bran, corn bran,
rice bran, whole-grain cereals and breads, dried beans and peas, nuts,
seeds, and the skins of fruits and vegetables. Foods containing insoluble
fiber have been shown to promote bowel regularity and may prevent
constipation, diverticulosis, and hemorrhoids.

Soluble fibers will dissolve in water and form a gel, which slows both
the stomach emptying time and the absorption of sugars from the
intestines. Your best sources of soluble fiber are fruits and vegetables,
oat bran, barley, dried beans and peas, psyllium, and flax seed. Foods
high in soluble fiber have been associated with lowering blood cholesterol levels and helping to regulate blood sugar levels for people with
type 2 diabetes. In addition, soluble fiber may also help with weight
control since it slows the emptying of the stomach, helping you to feel
fuller for longer.

Most people do not eat enough fiber. The table on the facing page
shows the fiber content of many common foods. Try to eat foods that

FIBER CONTENT OF COMMON FOODS		
FOOD	**SERVING SIZE**	**GRAMS OF FIBER**
FRUITS		
Apple	1 medium	5.5
Banana	1 medium	2
Cherries	10	1.5
Grapefruit	1/2 medium	1
Grapes	1 1/2 cups	3
Nectarine	1 medium	2
Orange	1 medium	4
Pear	1 medium	4.5
Pineapple	2 slices	3
Strawberries	6 medium	1.5
VEGETABLES		
Asparagus	4 spears	2
Avocado	1/2 medium	3
Broccoli	1/2 cup cooked	2
Carrots	1 medium	2.7
Green beans	1/2 cup	2
Leaf lettuce	1 1/2 cups	1
Potato with skin	1 medium	4
Sweet potato with skin	1 medium	4
Tomato	1 medium	2
GRAINS		
All-Bran	1/2 cup	10
Bran muffin	1 small	2.5
Brown rice, cooked	1 cup	3.2
Cheerios (whole grain) cereal	3/4 cup	3
Popcorn, air-popped	3 cups	2
Wheaties Energy Crunch	1 cup	4
Whole wheat bread	1 slice	1.5
BEANS AND NUTS		
Baked beans	1/2 cup	10
Kidney beans	1/2 cup	7
Peanut butter, smooth	2 tablespoons	1.8
Peanuts, roasted	1 oz	2.5

contain 3 or more grams of fiber per serving, for a total of at least 25 to 35 grams of fiber each day.

Don't Skip Dairy

Many dieters avoid milk and other dairy products in an effort to avoid dietary fat. New research suggests that having an adequate intake of calcium may be important for maintaining a healthy weight. In general, body mass index (BMI) has been found to be higher in people with low calcium intake. This may be because calcium plays an important role in getting fat out of your fat cells. Research from our laboratory suggests that calcium may also help your body to burn fat rather than store it. Some studies have even shown that including low-fat dairy products helps with weight loss when used as part of a reasonable weight-loss program. Calcium is no magic bullet, but we all need calcium, and if it helps with weight management, all the better.

While we think calcium can help your weight, we *know* it can help your bones and your blood pressure. Because most people get too little calcium, we recommend that you do not eliminate low-fat dairy products from your diet. Try to choose skim milk and the low-fat or fat-free versions of other dairy products. The prevailing recommendation of three daily servings of dairy is not a bad one for weight management.

Low-fat sources of dairy include low-fat and skim milk, low-fat and fat-free yogurt, reduced-fat cheese, and low-fat and fat-free cottage cheese. Nondairy sources of calcium include canned salmon with bones, fortified cereals and juices, collards, kale, and spinach.

BodySteps Tables

The following tables allow you to calculate your BodySteps—the amount of energy your body uses up on its own. First find the correct table for your sex and your age. Next, find the BodyStep value that corresponds to your height at the top and your weight at the side. If your height or weight is not on the table, use the closest value of each. Now you know your BodyStep number, the number of steps your body burns for you.

ENERGY EXPENDITURE IN BODYSTEPS
Women Ages 20–25

Weight	Height 4'10"	4'11"	5'0"	5'1"	5'2"	5'3"	5'4"
100	49,839	49,178	48,538	47,920	47,321	46,742	46,180
105	48,287	47,643	47,020	46,418	45,836	45,271	44,725
110	46,875	46,247	45,640	45,053	44,485	43,935	43,402
115	45,586	44,973	44,380	43,807	43,252	42,714	42,194
120	44,405	43,805	43,225	42,664	42,121	41,596	41,086
125	43,318	42,730	42,162	41,613	41,081	40,566	40,068
130	42,315	41,738	41,181	40,643	40,121	39,616	39,127
135	41,386	40,820	40,273	39,744	39,232	38,737	38,256
140	40,523	39,967	39,430	38,910	38,407	37,920	37,448
145	39,720	39,173	38,644	38,133	37,638	37,159	36,695
150	38,970	38,432	37,912	37,408	36,921	36,449	35,992
155	38,269	37,739	37,226	36,730	36,250	35,785	35,335
160	37,612	37,089	36,583	36,094	35,621	35,163	34,719
165	36,994	36,478	35,979	35,497	35,030	34,578	34,140
170	36,413	35,904	35,411	34,935	34,474	34,028	33,595
175	35,865	35,362	34,875	34,405	33,950	33,509	33,082
180	35,347	34,850	34,369	33,904	33,454	33,019	32,597
185	34,858	34,366	33,891	33,431	32,986	32,555	32,138
190	34,394	33,907	33,437	32,982	32,542	32,116	31,703
195	33,954	33,472	33,007	32,557	32,121	31,699	31,290
200	33,536	33,059	32,598	32,152	31,721	31,303	30,899
205	33,138	32,666	32,209	31,768	31,340	30,927	30,526
210	32,760	32,292	31,839	31,402	30,978	30,568	30,171
215	32,398	31,935	31,486	31,052	30,633	30,226	29,832
220	32,054	31,594	31,149	30,719	30,303	29,900	29,509
225	31,724	31,268	30,827	30,400	29,988	29,588	29,201
230	31,409	30,957	30,519	30,096	29,686	29,290	28,905
235	31,108	30,658	30,224	29,804	29,398	29,004	28,623
240	30,819	30,373	29,942	29,524	29,121	28,730	28,352
245	30,541	30,099	29,670	29,256	28,856	28,468	28,092
250	30,275	29,835	29,410	28,999	28,601	28,216	27,842
255	30,019	29,583	29,160	28,752	28,356	27,973	27,603
260	29,774	29,339	28,920	28,514	28,121	27,741	27,372
265	29,537	29,105	28,688	28,285	27,894	27,516	27,150
270	29,309	28,880	28,466	28,065	27,676	27,301	26,937
275	29,090	28,663	28,251	27,852	27,466	27,093	26,731
280	28,878	28,454	28,044	27,647	27,264	26,892	26,532
285	28,673	28,252	27,844	27,450	27,068	26,699	26,341
290	28,476	28,057	27,651	27,259	26,879	26,512	26,156
295	28,286	27,868	27,465	27,075	26,697	26,332	25,977
300	28,101	27,686	27,285	26,897	26,521	26,157	25,805

ENERGY EXPENDITURE IN BODYSTEPS
Women Ages 20–25

5'5"	5'6"	5'7"	5'8"	5'9"	5'10"	5'11"	6'0"
45,636	45,108	44,596	44,100	43,617	43,148	42,693	42,250
44,195	43,681	43,183	42,699	42,230	41,774	41,330	40,899
42,885	42,384	41,898	41,427	40,969	40,524	40,091	39,671
41,689	41,200	40,725	40,265	39,817	39,383	38,960	38,550
40,593	40,114	39,650	39,199	38,762	38,337	37,924	37,522
39,584	39,115	38,661	38,219	37,791	37,374	36,970	36,576
38,653	38,193	37,747	37,315	36,894	36,486	36,089	35,703
37,791	37,340	36,902	36,477	36,064	35,664	35,274	34,895
36,991	36,547	36,117	35,699	35,294	34,900	34,517	34,145
36,245	35,809	35,386	34,975	34,576	34,189	33,812	33,446
35,550	35,120	34,703	34,299	33,906	33,525	33,154	32,794
34,899	34,476	34,065	33,667	33,280	32,904	32,539	32,184
34,289	33,872	33,467	33,074	32,693	32,322	31,962	31,612
33,716	33,304	32,905	32,517	32,141	31,775	31,420	31,075
33,176	32,770	32,376	31,993	31,622	31,261	30,910	30,569
32,668	32,266	31,877	31,499	31,132	30,775	30,429	30,092
32,187	31,791	31,406	31,032	30,670	30,317	29,975	29,642
31,733	31,341	30,960	30,591	30,232	29,884	29,545	29,216
31,303	30,915	30,538	30,173	29,818	29,473	29,138	28,812
30,894	30,510	30,138	29,776	29,425	29,083	28,752	28,430
30,506	30,126	29,757	29,399	29,051	28,713	28,385	28,066
30,137	29,761	29,395	29,040	28,696	28,361	28,036	27,720
29,786	29,413	29,050	28,699	28,358	28,026	27,704	27,390
29,451	29,081	28,722	28,373	28,035	27,706	27,387	27,076
29,131	28,764	28,408	28,062	27,727	27,401	27,084	26,776
28,825	28,461	28,108	27,765	27,433	27,109	26,795	26,490
28,533	28,172	27,821	27,481	27,151	26,830	26,519	26,216
28,253	27,895	27,547	27,209	26,882	26,563	26,254	25,953
27,985	27,629	27,284	26,949	26,623	26,307	26,000	25,702
27,727	27,374	27,031	26,699	26,376	26,062	25,757	25,461
27,480	27,130	26,789	26,459	26,138	25,826	25,523	25,229
27,243	26,895	26,556	26,228	25,909	25,600	25,299	25,007
27,015	26,669	26,333	26,006	25,690	25,382	25,083	24,793
26,795	26,451	26,117	25,793	25,478	25,173	24,876	24,587
26,584	26,242	25,910	25,588	25,275	24,971	24,676	24,388
26,380	26,040	25,710	25,390	25,079	24,776	24,483	24,197
26,184	25,845	25,517	25,199	24,889	24,589	24,297	24,013
25,994	25,658	25,331	25,014	24,707	24,408	24,118	23,835
25,811	25,476	25,152	24,837	24,531	24,233	23,945	23,664
25,634	25,301	24,978	24,665	24,360	24,065	23,777	23,498
25,463	25,132	24,811	24,499	24,196	23,902	23,616	23,338

ENERGY EXPENDITURE IN BODYSTEPS
Women Ages 26–30

Weight	Height 4'10"	4'11"	5'0"	5'1"	5'2"	5'3"	5'4"
100	48,819	48,174	47,552	46,949	46,366	45,802	45,255
105	47,315	46,687	46,081	45,494	44,926	44,376	43,844
110	45,947	45,335	44,743	44,171	43,617	43,080	42,561
115	44,699	44,100	43,522	42,963	42,421	41,897	41,389
120	43,554	42,969	42,403	41,855	41,325	40,812	40,315
125	42,501	41,928	41,373	40,836	40,317	39,815	39,328
130	41,530	40,967	40,422	39,896	39,387	38,893	38,416
135	40,630	40,077	39,542	39,025	38,525	38,040	37,571
140	39,794	39,250	38,725	38,217	37,725	37,248	36,787
145	39,016	38,481	37,964	37,464	36,980	36,511	36,057
150	38,290	37,763	37,254	36,761	36,284	35,823	35,376
155	37,611	37,091	36,589	36,104	35,634	35,179	34,738
160	36,974	36,462	35,967	35,488	35,024	34,576	34,141
165	36,376	35,870	35,381	34,909	34,451	34,009	33,579
170	35,813	35,313	34,831	34,364	33,912	33,475	33,051
175	35,282	34,788	34,312	33,850	33,404	32,972	32,553
180	34,780	34,293	33,821	33,365	32,924	32,497	32,083
185	34,306	33,824	33,357	32,906	32,470	32,047	31,638
190	33,857	33,379	32,918	32,471	32,039	31,621	31,216
195	33,431	32,958	32,501	32,059	31,631	31,217	30,816
200	33,026	32,557	32,105	31,667	31,244	30,833	30,436
205	32,640	32,176	31,728	31,294	30,875	30,468	30,075
210	32,274	31,814	31,369	30,939	30,523	30,121	29,730
215	31,924	31,468	31,027	30,601	30,188	29,789	29,402
220	31,590	31,138	30,701	30,278	29,869	29,473	29,089
225	31,271	30,822	30,389	29,969	29,563	29,170	28,789
230	30,966	30,520	30,090	29,674	29,271	28,881	28,503
235	30,673	30,231	29,804	29,391	28,991	28,604	28,229
240	30,393	29,955	29,530	29,120	28,723	28,339	27,966
245	30,125	29,689	29,268	28,860	28,466	28,084	27,714
250	29,867	29,434	29,015	28,611	28,219	27,840	27,472
255	29,619	29,189	28,773	28,371	27,982	27,605	27,240
260	29,381	28,953	28,540	28,140	27,754	27,379	27,016
265	29,152	28,727	28,316	27,919	27,534	27,162	26,801
270	28,931	28,509	28,100	27,705	27,323	26,953	26,594
275	28,718	28,298	27,892	27,499	27,119	26,751	26,394
280	28,513	28,095	27,691	27,301	26,923	26,557	26,202
285	28,315	27,900	27,498	27,109	26,733	26,369	26,016
290	28,124	27,711	27,311	26,924	26,550	26,188	25,837
295	27,940	27,528	27,130	26,746	26,373	26,013	25,664
300	27,761	27,352	26,956	26,573	26,203	25,844	25,496

APPENDIX B

ENERGY EXPENDITURE IN BODYSTEPS
Women Ages 26–30

5'5"	5'6"	5'7"	5'8"	5'9"	5'10"	5'11"	6'0"
44,725	44,211	43,713	43,229	42,759	42,303	41,859	41,428
43,328	42,827	42,342	41,870	41,413	40,968	40,536	40,116
42,057	41,569	41,095	40,635	40,189	39,755	39,333	38,924
40,897	40,420	39,957	39,507	39,071	38,647	38,235	37,835
39,834	39,367	38,914	38,474	38,047	37,632	37,229	36,837
38,856	38,398	37,954	37,523	37,104	36,698	36,303	35,919
37,952	37,503	37,068	36,645	36,234	35,835	35,448	35,071
37,116	36,675	36,247	35,832	35,429	35,037	34,656	34,286
36,340	35,906	35,486	35,077	34,681	34,296	33,921	33,557
35,617	35,190	34,776	34,375	33,984	33,605	33,237	32,879
34,942	34,522	34,114	33,719	33,334	32,961	32,598	32,246
34,311	33,897	33,495	33,105	32,726	32,358	32,001	31,653
33,720	33,311	32,915	32,530	32,156	31,793	31,441	31,098
33,164	32,760	32,369	31,990	31,621	31,263	30,915	30,576
32,641	32,242	31,856	31,481	31,117	30,763	30,419	30,085
32,147	31,754	31,372	31,001	30,642	30,292	29,953	29,622
31,681	31,292	30,915	30,549	30,193	29,847	29,512	29,185
31,241	30,856	30,483	30,120	29,768	29,427	29,094	28,771
30,823	30,442	30,073	29,714	29,366	29,028	28,699	28,380
30,427	30,050	29,684	29,329	28,985	28,650	28,324	28,008
30,051	29,677	29,315	28,964	28,622	28,290	27,968	27,655
29,693	29,323	28,964	28,616	28,277	27,949	27,629	27,319
29,352	28,985	28,630	28,284	27,949	27,623	27,307	26,999
29,027	28,664	28,311	27,968	27,636	27,313	26,999	26,694
28,717	28,356	28,006	27,667	27,337	27,017	26,705	26,403
28,420	28,063	27,715	27,379	27,051	26,734	26,425	26,124
28,137	27,782	27,437	27,103	26,778	26,463	26,156	25,858
27,865	27,513	27,171	26,839	26,517	26,204	25,899	25,603
27,605	27,255	26,916	26,586	26,266	25,955	25,653	25,359
27,356	27,008	26,671	26,343	26,026	25,717	25,417	25,125
27,116	26,771	26,436	26,110	25,795	25,488	25,190	24,900
26,886	26,543	26,210	25,887	25,573	25,268	24,972	24,684
26,665	26,324	25,993	25,672	25,360	25,057	24,762	24,476
26,452	26,113	25,784	25,465	25,155	24,853	24,561	24,276
26,246	25,909	25,582	25,265	24,957	24,658	24,367	24,084
26,049	25,714	25,389	25,073	24,767	24,469	24,180	23,898
25,858	25,525	25,202	24,888	24,583	24,287	23,999	23,720
25,674	25,343	25,021	24,709	24,406	24,111	23,825	23,547
25,497	25,167	24,847	24,536	24,235	23,942	23,657	23,380
25,325	24,997	24,679	24,370	24,070	23,778	23,495	23,219
25,159	24,833	24,516	24,208	23,910	23,620	23,338	23,064

ENERGY EXPENDITURE IN BODYSTEPS
Women Ages 31–35

Weight	Height 4'10"	4'11"	5'0"	5'1"	5'2"	5'3"	5'4"
100	47,891	47,262	46,655	46,067	45,498	44,948	44,414
105	46,431	45,818	45,226	44,654	44,099	43,563	43,043
110	45,104	44,506	43,928	43,369	42,828	42,304	41,796
115	43,892	43,307	42,742	42,195	41,666	41,154	40,658
120	42,781	42,209	41,655	41,120	40,602	40,101	39,615
125	41,759	41,198	40,655	40,131	39,623	39,131	38,655
130	40,816	40,265	39,732	39,217	38,719	38,236	37,769
135	39,942	39,401	38,878	38,372	37,882	37,408	36,948
140	39,131	38,599	38,084	37,586	37,105	36,638	36,186
145	38,376	37,852	37,345	36,855	36,381	35,922	35,477
150	37,671	37,155	36,656	36,173	35,706	35,253	34,815
155	37,012	36,503	36,011	35,535	35,074	34,628	34,196
160	36,394	35,892	35,406	34,936	34,482	34,042	33,615
165	35,813	35,317	34,838	34,374	33,925	33,491	33,070
170	35,267	34,777	34,303	33,845	33,402	32,972	32,556
175	34,751	34,267	33,799	33,346	32,908	32,484	32,073
180	34,265	33,786	33,323	32,875	32,442	32,022	31,615
185	33,804	33,331	32,872	32,429	32,000	31,585	31,183
190	33,368	32,899	32,446	32,007	31,583	31,172	30,773
195	32,955	32,490	32,041	31,606	31,186	30,779	30,385
200	32,562	32,101	31,656	31,226	30,809	30,406	30,016
205	32,188	31,732	31,291	30,864	30,451	30,052	29,664
210	31,832	31,379	30,942	30,519	30,110	29,714	29,330
215	30,007	29,574	30,610	30,191	29,785	29,392	29,011
220	31,168	30,723	30,293	29,877	29,474	29,084	28,707
225	30,858	30,417	29,990	29,577	29,177	28,791	28,416
230	30,562	30,124	29,700	29,290	28,894	28,510	28,137
235	30,279	29,843	29,423	29,016	28,622	28,240	27,871
240	30,007	29,574	29,157	28,752	28,361	27,983	27,616
245	29,746	29,317	28,902	28,500	28,112	27,735	27,371
250	29,496	29,069	28,657	28,258	27,872	27,498	27,136
255	29,255	28,831	28,421	28,025	27,641	27,270	26,910
260	29,024	28,603	28,195	27,801	27,420	27,050	26,693
265	28,802	28,383	27,977	27,586	27,207	26,839	26,484
270	28,587	28,171	27,768	27,378	27,001	26,636	26,283
275	28,381	27,966	27,566	27,178	26,803	26,440	26,089
280	28,182	27,770	27,371	26,986	26,613	26,252	25,902
285	27,990	27,580	27,183	26,800	26,429	26,069	25,721
290	27,804	27,396	27,002	26,620	26,251	25,893	25,547
295	27,625	27,219	26,826	26,447	26,079	25,723	25,379
300	27,452	27,048	26,657	26,279	25,913	25,559	25,216

ENERGY EXPENDITURE IN BODYSTEPS
Women Ages 31–35

5'5"	5'6"	5'7"	5'8"	5'9"	5'10"	5'11"	6'0"
43,897	43,396	42,909	42,437	41,979	41,534	41,101	40,680
42,539	42,051	41,577	41,116	40,670	40,236	39,814	39,404
41,304	40,827	40,365	39,916	39,480	39,056	38,644	38,244
40,177	39,711	39,258	38,819	38,393	37,979	37,576	37,185
39,144	38,687	38,244	37,814	37,397	36,991	36,597	36,214
38,193	37,745	37,311	36,890	36,480	36,083	35,696	35,320
37,316	36,876	36,450	36,036	35,634	35,244	34,865	34,496
36,503	36,071	35,652	35,246	34,851	34,467	34,095	33,732
35,748	35,324	34,912	34,512	34,124	33,746	33,380	33,023
35,046	34,628	34,222	33,829	33,446	33,075	32,714	32,363
34,390	33,978	33,579	33,191	32,814	32,449	32,093	31,747
33,777	33,371	32,977	32,594	32,223	31,862	31,512	31,171
33,202	32,801	32,413	32,035	31,669	31,313	30,967	30,631
32,662	32,266	31,882	31,510	31,148	30,797	30,455	30,123
32,153	31,763	31,383	31,015	30,658	30,311	29,974	29,646
31,674	31,288	30,913	30,549	30,196	29,853	29,519	29,195
31,221	30,839	30,469	30,109	29,760	29,420	29,090	28,770
30,793	30,415	30,048	29,692	29,347	29,011	28,685	28,367
30,387	30,013	29,650	29,298	28,956	28,623	28,300	27,986
30,003	29,632	29,272	28,923	28,585	28,255	27,936	27,625
29,637	29,270	28,914	28,568	28,232	27,906	27,589	27,281
29,289	28,925	28,572	28,230	27,897	27,574	27,260	26,954
28,958	28,597	28,247	27,907	27,577	27,257	26,946	26,643
28,642	28,284	27,937	27,600	27,273	26,955	26,646	26,346
28,341	27,986	27,641	27,307	26,982	26,667	26,361	26,063
28,052	27,700	27,358	27,027	26,705	26,392	26,088	25,792
27,777	27,427	27,088	26,759	26,439	26,128	25,827	25,533
27,513	27,166	26,829	26,502	26,185	25,876	25,577	25,285
27,260	26,915	26,581	26,256	25,941	25,635	25,337	25,048
27,018	26,675	26,343	26,020	25,707	25,403	25,107	24,820
26,785	26,445	26,114	25,794	25,483	25,180	24,887	24,601
26,561	26,223	25,895	25,576	25,267	24,967	24,675	24,391
26,346	26,010	25,684	25,367	25,060	24,761	24,471	24,189
26,139	25,805	25,481	25,166	24,860	24,563	24,275	23,994
25,940	25,607	25,285	24,972	24,668	24,373	24,086	23,807
25,748	25,417	25,096	24,785	24,483	24,189	23,904	23,627
25,563	25,234	24,915	24,605	24,304	24,012	23,729	23,453
25,384	25,057	24,739	24,431	24,132	23,842	23,559	23,285
25,211	24,886	24,570	24,263	23,966	23,677	23,396	23,123
25,045	24,721	24,406	24,101	23,805	23,517	23,238	22,966
24,883	24,561	24,248	23,945	23,650	23,363	23,085	22,815

ENERGY EXPENDITURE IN BODYSTEPS
Women Ages 36–40

Weight	Height 4'10"	4'11"	5'0"	5'1"	5'2"	5'3"	5'4"
100	46,963	45,758	45,758	45,185	44,630	44,093	43,573
105	45,547	44,950	44,372	43,813	43,273	42,749	42,242
110	44,260	43,676	43,112	42,567	42,038	41,527	41,032
115	43,085	42,514	41,962	41,428	40,912	40,411	39,927
120	42,008	41,448	40,908	40,385	39,879	39,389	38,914
125	41,017	40,468	39,938	39,425	38,928	38,448	37,982
130	40,102	39,563	39,042	38,539	38,051	37,579	37,122
135	39,255	38,725	38,213	37,718	37,239	36,775	36,325
140	38,468	37,947	37,443	36,956	36,485	36,028	35,586
145	37,736	37,223	36,727	36,247	35,782	35,333	34,897
150	37,053	36,547	36,058	35,585	35,127	34,684	34,254
155	36,413	35,914	35,432	34,965	34,514	34,077	33,653
160	35,814	35,321	34,845	34,385	33,939	33,508	33,090
165	35,251	34,764	34,294	33,839	33,399	32,973	32,560
170	34,721	34,240	33,775	33,326	32,891	32,470	32,062
175	34,221	33,746	33,286	32,842	32,412	31,995	31,592
180	33,749	33,279	32,824	32,385	31,959	31,547	31,148
185	33,303	32,837	32,388	31,952	31,531	31,123	30,728
190	32,880	32,419	31,974	31,543	31,126	30,722	30,331
195	32,479	32,022	31,581	31,154	30,741	30,341	29,953
200	32,098	31,645	31,208	30,785	30,375	29,979	29,595
205	31,735	31,287	30,853	30,434	30,028	29,635	29,254
210	31,390	30,945	30,515	30,099	29,697	29,307	28,929
215	28,451	28,038	30,193	29,780	29,381	28,994	28,620
220	30,746	30,308	29,885	29,476	29,080	28,696	28,324
225	30,446	30,011	29,591	29,185	28,792	28,411	28,042
230	30,159	29,727	29,310	28,907	28,516	28,138	27,772
235	29,884	29,455	29,041	28,640	28,252	27,877	27,513
240	28,451	28,038	28,783	28,385	28,000	27,627	27,265
245	29,367	28,944	28,535	28,140	27,757	27,387	27,028
250	29,125	28,704	28,298	27,905	27,524	27,156	26,799
255	28,891	28,474	28,070	27,679	27,301	26,935	26,580
260	28,667	28,252	27,850	27,462	27,086	26,722	26,369
265	28,451	28,038	27,639	27,253	26,879	26,517	26,166
270	28,244	27,833	27,436	27,052	26,680	26,320	25,971
275	28,043	27,635	27,240	26,858	26,488	26,130	25,783
280	27,850	27,444	27,051	26,671	26,303	25,946	25,601
285	27,664	27,260	26,868	26,490	26,124	25,770	25,426
290	27,484	27,082	26,692	26,316	25,952	25,599	25,257
295	27,311	26,910	26,522	26,148	25,785	25,434	25,094
300	27,143	26,744	26,358	25,985	25,624	25,274	24,936

ENERGY EXPENDITURE IN BODYSTEPS
Women Ages 36–40

5'5"	5'6"	5'7"	5'8"	5'9"	5'10"	5'11"	6'0"
43,069	42,580	42,106	41,646	41,199	40,765	40,343	39,933
41,750	41,274	40,811	40,363	39,927	39,504	39,092	38,692
40,552	40,086	39,634	39,196	38,770	38,357	37,955	37,564
39,457	39,002	38,560	38,131	37,715	37,310	36,917	36,535
38,454	38,008	37,575	37,155	36,747	36,350	35,965	35,591
37,531	37,093	36,668	36,256	35,856	35,468	35,090	34,722
36,679	36,249	35,832	35,427	35,034	34,653	34,282	33,921
35,890	35,467	35,057	34,659	34,273	33,898	33,533	33,179
35,157	34,741	34,338	33,947	33,566	33,197	32,838	32,490
34,475	34,066	33,668	33,283	32,908	32,545	32,191	31,848
33,838	33,435	33,043	32,663	32,294	31,936	31,588	31,249
33,243	32,845	32,459	32,084	31,720	31,366	31,023	30,689
32,684	32,292	31,910	31,541	31,181	30,832	30,493	30,164
32,160	31,772	31,396	31,030	30,675	30,331	29,996	29,670
31,666	31,283	30,911	30,550	30,199	29,859	29,528	29,206
31,201	30,822	30,454	30,097	29,750	29,413	29,086	28,768
30,761	30,386	30,022	29,669	29,326	28,993	28,669	28,354
30,346	29,974	29,614	29,265	28,925	28,595	28,275	27,963
29,952	29,584	29,227	28,881	28,545	28,219	27,901	27,593
29,578	29,214	28,860	28,518	28,185	27,861	27,547	27,241
29,223	28,862	28,512	28,172	27,842	27,522	27,210	26,907
28,885	28,527	28,180	27,843	27,516	27,199	26,890	26,589
28,564	28,209	27,865	27,530	27,206	26,891	26,585	26,287
28,257	27,905	27,563	27,232	26,910	26,598	26,294	25,998
27,964	27,615	27,276	26,947	26,628	26,318	26,016	25,723
27,684	27,338	27,001	26,675	26,358	26,050	25,751	25,460
27,417	27,073	26,739	26,415	26,100	25,794	25,497	25,208
27,161	26,819	26,487	26,165	25,853	25,549	25,254	24,967
26,915	26,576	26,246	25,926	25,616	25,314	25,021	24,736
26,680	26,342	26,015	25,697	25,389	25,089	24,798	24,515
26,454	26,118	25,793	25,477	25,171	24,873	24,583	24,302
26,236	25,903	25,580	25,266	24,961	24,665	24,377	24,098
26,028	25,696	25,375	25,063	24,760	24,465	24,179	23,901
25,827	25,497	25,177	24,867	24,566	24,273	23,989	23,712
25,633	25,305	24,987	24,679	24,379	24,088	23,805	23,530
25,447	25,121	24,804	24,497	24,199	23,910	23,628	23,355
25,267	24,942	24,628	24,322	24,026	23,738	23,458	23,186
25,093	24,771	24,457	24,154	23,858	23,572	23,293	23,022
24,926	24,605	24,293	23,991	23,697	23,412	23,134	22,865
24,764	24,444	24,134	23,833	23,541	23,257	22,981	22,713
24,607	24,289	23,980	23,681	23,390	23,107	22,832	22,565

ENERGY EXPENDITURE IN BODYSTEPS
Women Ages 41–45

Weight	Height 4'10"	4'11"	5'0"	5'1"	5'2"	5'3"	5'4"
100	46,035	45,438	44,861	44,302	43,762	43,239	42,732
105	44,663	44,081	43,518	42,973	42,446	41,936	41,441
110	43,416	42,847	42,297	41,764	41,249	40,750	40,267
115	42,278	41,721	41,182	40,661	40,157	39,668	39,196
120	41,234	40,688	40,160	39,649	39,155	38,677	38,213
125	40,274	39,738	39,220	38,719	38,234	37,764	37,309
130	39,388	38,861	38,352	37,860	37,383	36,922	36,475
135	38,568	38,050	37,549	37,065	36,596	36,142	35,702
140	37,806	37,296	36,803	36,326	35,865	35,418	34,985
145	37,096	36,594	36,108	35,638	35,184	34,744	34,317
150	36,434	35,939	35,460	34,997	34,548	34,114	33,694
155	35,815	35,326	34,853	34,396	33,954	33,526	33,111
160	35,234	34,751	34,285	33,833	33,397	32,974	32,564
165	34,688	34,212	33,750	33,305	32,873	32,455	32,050
170	34,175	33,704	33,248	32,807	32,380	31,967	31,567
175	33,691	33,225	32,774	32,338	31,916	31,507	31,111
180	33,234	32,772	32,326	31,895	31,477	31,073	30,681
185	32,801	32,344	31,903	31,475	31,062	30,662	30,274
190	32,392	31,939	31,501	31,078	30,669	30,272	29,888
195	32,003	31,554	31,121	30,702	30,296	29,903	29,522
200	31,634	31,189	30,759	30,344	29,941	29,552	29,175
205	31,282	30,842	30,415	30,003	29,604	29,218	28,844
210	30,948	30,511	30,088	29,679	29,283	28,900	28,529
215	27,164	26,767	29,775	29,370	28,977	28,597	28,229
220	30,324	29,894	29,477	29,075	28,685	28,308	27,942
225	30,033	29,606	29,192	28,793	28,406	28,031	27,668
230	29,755	29,331	28,920	28,523	28,139	27,767	27,406
235	29,489	29,067	28,659	28,265	27,883	27,513	27,155
240	27,164	26,767	28,409	28,017	27,638	27,271	26,915
245	28,989	28,572	28,169	27,780	27,403	27,038	26,684
250	28,753	28,339	27,939	27,552	27,177	26,814	26,463
255	28,527	28,116	27,718	27,333	26,960	26,600	26,250
260	28,310	27,901	27,505	27,122	26,752	26,393	26,046
265	27,164	26,767	27,300	26,920	26,551	26,195	25,849
270	27,900	27,495	27,103	26,725	26,358	26,003	25,660
275	27,706	27,303	26,913	26,537	26,172	25,819	25,477
280	27,519	27,118	26,730	26,355	25,993	25,641	25,301
285	27,339	26,939	26,554	26,181	25,819	25,470	25,131
290	27,164	26,767	26,383	26,012	25,652	25,304	24,967
295	26,996	26,600	26,218	25,848	25,491	25,144	24,809
300	26,833	26,439	26,059	25,691	25,334	24,990	24,655

ENERGY EXPENDITURE IN BODYSTEPS
Women Ages 41–45

5'5"	5'6"	5'7"	5'8"	5'9"	5'10"	5'11"	6'0"
42,241	41,765	41,303	40,854	40,419	39,996	39,585	39,185
40,962	40,497	40,046	39,609	39,184	38,771	38,370	37,980
39,799	39,345	38,904	38,477	38,061	37,658	37,266	36,885
38,737	38,293	37,861	37,443	37,036	36,641	36,258	35,885
37,764	37,328	36,905	36,495	36,097	35,710	35,334	34,968
36,868	36,441	36,026	35,623	35,232	34,852	34,483	34,124
36,042	35,622	35,214	34,818	34,434	34,061	33,698	33,346
35,276	34,863	34,462	34,073	33,695	33,328	32,972	32,625
34,566	34,159	33,764	33,381	33,009	32,648	32,297	31,956
33,904	33,503	33,114	32,737	32,371	32,015	31,669	31,332
33,286	32,891	32,508	32,136	31,774	31,423	31,082	30,751
32,709	32,319	31,940	31,573	31,217	30,870	30,534	30,207
32,167	31,782	31,408	31,046	30,694	30,352	30,019	29,696
31,658	31,278	30,909	30,550	30,203	29,865	29,536	29,217
31,179	30,803	30,438	30,084	29,740	29,406	29,082	28,766
30,728	30,356	29,995	29,645	29,304	28,974	28,653	28,341
30,301	29,933	29,576	29,229	28,893	28,566	28,248	27,939
29,898	29,534	29,180	28,837	28,503	28,180	27,865	27,559
29,516	29,155	28,805	28,465	28,135	27,814	27,502	27,199
29,153	28,796	28,449	28,112	27,785	27,467	27,158	26,858
28,809	28,454	28,110	27,776	27,452	27,137	26,831	26,533
28,481	28,130	27,788	27,457	27,136	26,823	26,520	26,225
28,169	27,820	27,482	27,154	26,835	26,525	26,224	25,931
27,872	27,526	27,190	26,864	26,547	26,240	25,941	25,651
27,588	27,244	26,911	26,587	26,273	25,968	25,672	25,383
27,316	26,975	26,644	26,323	26,011	25,708	25,414	25,128
27,057	26,718	26,389	26,070	25,761	25,460	25,167	24,883
26,808	26,472	26,145	25,829	25,521	25,222	24,932	24,649
26,570	26,236	25,911	25,597	25,291	24,994	24,705	24,425
26,342	26,009	25,687	25,374	25,070	24,775	24,488	24,210
26,122	25,792	25,472	25,161	24,859	24,565	24,280	24,003
25,912	25,583	25,265	24,956	24,655	24,364	24,080	23,805
25,709	25,383	25,066	24,758	24,460	24,170	23,888	23,614
25,514	25,189	24,874	24,568	24,272	23,983	23,703	23,430
25,326	25,003	24,690	24,386	24,090	23,803	23,524	23,253
25,146	24,824	24,512	24,210	23,916	23,630	23,353	23,083
24,971	24,651	24,341	24,040	23,747	23,463	23,187	22,919
24,803	24,484	24,176	23,876	23,585	23,302	23,027	22,760
24,640	24,323	24,016	23,718	23,428	23,146	22,873	22,607
24,483	24,168	23,862	23,565	23,276	22,996	22,724	22,459
24,331	24,017	23,713	23,417	23,130	22,851	22,580	22,316

ENERGY EXPENDITURE IN BODYSTEPS
Women Ages 46–50

Weight	Height 4'10"	4'11"	5'0"	5'1"	5'2"	5'3"	5'4"
100	45,107	44,526	43,964	43,420	42,894	42,385	41,891
105	43,780	43,212	42,663	42,133	41,619	41,122	40,640
110	42,573	42,018	41,481	40,962	40,460	39,974	39,503
115	41,471	40,927	40,402	39,894	39,402	38,926	38,464
120	40,461	39,928	39,413	38,914	38,432	37,965	37,512
125	39,532	39,008	38,502	38,013	37,539	37,081	36,636
130	38,674	38,160	37,662	37,181	36,716	36,265	35,828
135	37,880	37,374	36,884	36,411	35,953	35,509	35,079
140	37,143	36,644	36,162	35,696	35,244	34,808	34,384
145	36,456	35,965	35,489	35,030	34,585	34,154	33,737
150	35,815	35,330	34,862	34,408	33,970	33,545	33,133
155	35,216	34,737	34,275	33,827	33,394	32,974	32,568
160	34,654	34,181	33,724	33,282	32,854	32,440	32,038
165	34,126	33,659	33,207	32,770	32,347	31,937	31,541
170	33,629	33,167	32,720	32,288	31,870	31,465	31,072
175	33,161	32,703	32,261	31,834	31,420	31,019	30,631
180	32,718	32,265	31,828	31,404	30,995	30,598	30,214
185	32,300	31,851	31,418	30,999	30,593	30,200	29,819
190	31,903	31,459	31,029	30,614	30,212	29,823	29,446
195	31,527	31,087	30,661	30,249	29,851	29,465	29,091
200	31,170	30,733	30,311	29,902	29,507	29,125	28,754
205	30,830	30,397	29,978	29,573	29,181	28,801	28,434
210	30,506	30,076	29,661	29,259	28,870	28,493	28,129
215	30,197	29,771	29,358	28,959	28,573	28,200	27,838
220	29,903	29,479	29,070	28,674	28,290	27,919	27,560
225	29,621	29,200	28,794	28,401	28,020	27,651	27,294
230	29,352	28,934	28,530	28,139	27,761	27,395	27,041
235	29,094	28,679	28,277	27,889	27,514	27,150	26,798
240	28,847	28,434	28,035	27,650	27,276	26,915	26,565
245	28,610	28,200	27,803	27,420	27,049	26,689	26,341
250	28,382	27,974	27,580	27,199	26,830	26,473	26,127
255	28,164	27,758	27,366	26,987	26,620	26,265	25,921
260	27,953	27,550	27,160	26,783	26,418	26,065	25,722
265	27,751	27,350	26,962	26,587	26,224	25,872	25,532
270	27,556	27,157	26,771	26,398	26,037	25,687	25,348
275	27,369	26,971	26,587	26,216	25,856	25,508	25,171
280	27,188	26,792	26,410	26,040	25,683	25,336	25,001
285	27,013	26,619	26,239	25,871	25,515	25,170	24,836
290	26,844	26,452	26,074	25,707	25,353	25,010	24,677
295	26,681	26,291	25,914	25,549	25,196	24,855	24,523
300	26,524	26,135	25,760	25,397	25,045	24,705	24,375

ENERGY EXPENDITURE IN BODYSTEPS
Women Ages 46–50

5'5"	5'6"	5'7"	5'8"	5'9"	5'10"	5'11"	6'0"
41,413	40,949	40,500	40,063	39,639	39,227	38,827	38,438
40,173	39,721	39,281	38,855	38,441	38,039	37,648	37,268
39,046	38,603	38,174	37,757	37,352	36,959	36,577	36,205
38,017	37,583	37,163	36,754	36,358	35,973	35,599	35,235
37,074	36,648	36,236	35,835	35,447	35,069	34,702	34,345
36,206	35,788	35,383	34,990	34,608	34,237	33,877	33,526
35,405	34,994	34,596	34,210	33,834	33,470	33,115	32,771
34,663	34,259	33,867	33,487	33,118	32,759	32,410	32,071
33,974	33,576	33,190	32,816	32,452	32,099	31,755	31,422
33,333	32,941	32,560	32,191	31,833	31,484	31,146	30,817
32,734	32,347	31,972	31,608	31,254	30,911	30,577	30,252
32,174	31,793	31,422	31,063	30,713	30,374	30,045	29,724
31,649	31,272	30,906	30,551	30,206	29,871	29,546	29,229
31,156	30,784	30,422	30,071	29,730	29,399	29,077	28,764
30,692	30,324	29,966	29,619	29,282	28,954	28,636	28,326
30,255	29,890	29,536	29,192	28,859	28,535	28,220	27,914
29,841	29,480	29,130	28,790	28,460	28,139	27,827	27,524
29,450	29,093	28,746	28,409	28,082	27,764	27,455	27,155
29,080	28,726	28,382	28,048	27,724	27,409	27,103	26,806
28,729	28,377	28,037	27,706	27,385	27,073	26,769	26,474
28,395	28,047	27,709	27,381	27,062	26,753	26,452	26,160
28,077	27,732	27,397	27,071	26,755	26,448	26,150	25,860
27,775	27,432	27,099	26,777	26,463	26,159	25,863	25,575
27,487	27,146	26,816	26,496	26,185	25,882	25,589	25,303
27,211	26,874	26,546	26,228	25,919	25,619	25,327	25,043
26,948	26,613	26,287	25,971	25,665	25,367	25,077	24,795
26,697	26,364	26,040	25,726	25,422	25,126	24,838	24,558
26,456	26,125	25,804	25,492	25,189	24,895	24,609	24,331
26,225	25,896	25,577	25,267	24,966	24,674	24,390	24,113
26,004	25,677	25,359	25,051	24,752	24,461	24,179	23,905
25,791	25,466	25,150	24,844	24,547	24,258	23,977	23,704
25,587	25,264	24,950	24,645	24,349	24,062	23,783	23,511
25,391	25,069	24,757	24,454	24,160	23,874	23,596	23,326
25,202	24,882	24,571	24,270	23,977	23,693	23,417	23,148
25,020	24,701	24,392	24,093	23,801	23,519	23,244	22,976
24,844	24,528	24,220	23,922	23,632	23,351	23,077	22,811
24,675	24,360	24,054	23,757	23,469	23,189	22,916	22,652
24,512	24,198	23,894	23,598	23,311	23,032	22,761	22,498
24,355	24,042	23,739	23,445	23,159	22,881	22,612	22,349
24,203	23,891	23,589	23,296	23,012	22,736	22,467	22,206
24,055	23,746	23,445	23,153	22,870	22,595	22,327	22,067

ENERGY EXPENDITURE IN BODYSTEPS
Women Ages 51–55

Weight	Height 4'10"	4'11"	5'0"	5'1"	5'2"	5'3"	5'4"
100	44,179	43,613	43,067	42,538	42,026	41,530	41,050
105	42,896	42,343	41,809	41,292	40,792	40,308	39,839
110	41,729	41,188	40,666	40,160	39,671	39,197	38,738
115	40,664	40,134	39,622	39,126	38,647	38,183	37,733
120	39,688	39,168	38,665	38,179	37,708	37,253	36,811
125	38,790	38,279	37,785	37,307	36,845	36,397	35,964
130	37,960	37,458	36,972	36,502	36,048	35,608	35,181
135	37,193	36,698	36,220	35,757	35,310	34,876	34,457
140	36,480	35,992	35,521	35,065	34,624	34,197	33,784
145	35,816	35,335	34,871	34,421	33,986	33,565	33,157
150	35,197	34,722	34,264	33,820	33,391	32,975	32,573
155	34,617	34,149	33,696	33,258	32,834	32,423	32,026
160	34,074	33,611	33,163	32,730	32,311	31,906	31,513
165	33,564	33,106	32,663	32,235	31,821	31,420	31,031
170	33,083	32,630	32,192	31,769	31,359	30,962	30,578
175	32,630	32,182	31,749	31,329	30,924	30,531	30,150
180	32,203	31,759	31,329	30,914	30,512	30,123	29,747
185	31,798	31,358	30,933	30,522	30,124	29,738	29,365
190	31,415	30,979	30,557	30,150	29,755	29,373	29,003
195	31,051	30,619	30,201	29,797	29,405	29,027	28,660
200	30,706	30,277	29,862	29,461	29,073	28,698	28,334
205	30,377	29,952	29,540	29,142	28,757	28,385	28,023
210	30,064	29,642	29,234	28,839	28,457	28,087	27,728
215	29,766	29,346	28,941	28,549	28,170	27,802	27,446
220	29,481	29,064	28,662	28,273	27,896	27,531	27,178
225	29,209	28,795	28,395	28,008	27,634	27,272	26,921
230	28,948	28,537	28,140	27,756	27,384	27,024	26,675
235	28,699	28,291	27,896	27,514	27,144	26,786	26,440
240	28,460	28,054	27,662	27,282	26,915	26,559	26,214
245	28,231	27,827	27,437	27,060	26,694	26,341	25,998
250	28,011	27,610	27,221	26,846	26,483	26,131	25,790
255	27,800	27,400	27,014	26,641	26,280	25,930	25,591
260	27,596	27,199	26,815	26,444	26,084	25,736	25,399
265	27,401	27,006	26,623	26,254	25,896	25,550	25,214
270	27,213	26,819	26,439	26,071	25,715	25,371	25,037
275	27,031	26,640	26,261	25,895	25,541	25,198	24,865
280	26,856	26,466	26,090	25,725	25,373	25,031	24,700
285	26,687	26,299	25,924	25,561	25,210	24,870	24,541
290	26,524	26,138	25,764	25,403	25,054	24,715	24,387
295	26,367	25,982	25,610	25,250	24,902	24,565	24,238
300	26,215	25,831	25,461	25,103	24,756	24,420	24,095

APPENDIX B

ENERGY EXPENDITURE IN BODYSTEPS
Women Ages 51–55

5'5"	5'6"	5'7"	5'8"	5'9"	5'10"	5'11"	6'0"
40,585	40,134	39,696	39,271	38,859	38,458	38,069	37,690
39,385	38,944	38,516	38,101	37,698	37,307	36,926	36,556
38,293	37,862	37,444	37,037	36,643	36,260	35,888	35,526
37,297	36,874	36,464	36,066	35,680	35,304	34,939	34,585
36,384	35,969	35,566	35,176	34,797	34,428	34,070	33,722
35,543	35,136	34,741	34,357	33,984	33,622	33,270	32,928
34,768	34,367	33,978	33,601	33,234	32,878	32,532	32,196
34,050	33,655	33,272	32,901	32,540	32,189	31,849	31,518
33,383	32,994	32,617	32,251	31,895	31,550	31,214	30,888
32,762	32,378	32,006	31,645	31,295	30,954	30,623	30,301
32,182	31,804	31,437	31,080	30,734	30,398	30,072	29,754
31,640	31,266	30,904	30,552	30,210	29,878	29,556	29,242
31,132	30,763	30,404	30,056	29,719	29,391	29,072	28,762
30,655	30,289	29,935	29,591	29,257	28,933	28,618	28,311
30,205	29,844	29,493	29,153	28,823	28,502	28,190	27,887
29,781	29,424	29,077	28,740	28,413	28,095	27,787	27,487
29,381	29,027	28,684	28,350	28,026	27,712	27,406	27,109
29,003	28,652	28,311	27,981	27,660	27,349	27,046	26,751
28,644	28,296	27,959	27,631	27,313	27,005	26,704	26,412
28,304	27,959	27,625	27,300	26,985	26,678	26,381	26,091
27,981	27,639	27,307	26,985	26,672	26,368	26,073	25,786
27,673	27,334	27,005	26,685	26,375	26,073	25,780	25,496
27,381	27,044	26,717	26,400	26,092	25,793	25,502	25,219
27,102	26,767	26,443	26,128	25,822	25,525	25,236	24,955
26,835	26,503	26,181	25,868	25,564	25,269	24,982	24,704
26,580	26,250	25,930	25,620	25,318	25,025	24,740	24,463
26,337	26,009	25,691	25,382	25,082	24,791	24,508	24,233
26,104	25,778	25,462	25,155	24,857	24,568	24,286	24,013
25,880	25,556	25,242	24,937	24,641	24,353	24,074	23,802
25,666	25,344	25,031	24,728	24,434	24,148	23,870	23,599
25,460	25,140	24,829	24,528	24,235	23,950	23,674	23,405
25,262	24,944	24,635	24,335	24,044	23,761	23,486	23,218
25,072	24,755	24,448	24,149	23,860	23,578	23,305	23,039
24,889	24,574	24,268	23,971	23,683	23,403	23,131	22,866
24,713	24,399	24,095	23,799	23,513	23,234	22,963	22,700
24,543	24,231	23,928	23,634	23,348	23,071	22,801	22,539
24,380	24,069	23,767	23,474	23,190	22,914	22,646	22,385
24,222	23,912	23,612	23,320	23,037	22,762	22,495	22,236
24,069	23,761	23,462	23,172	22,890	22,616	22,350	22,091
23,922	23,615	23,317	23,028	22,747	22,475	22,210	21,952
23,779	23,474	23,177	22,889	22,610	22,338	22,074	21,818

ENERGY EXPENDITURE IN BODYSTEPS
Women Ages 56–60

Weight	Height 4'10"	4'11"	5'0"	5'1"	5'2"	5'3"	5'4"
100	43,251	42,701	42,170	41,655	41,158	40,676	40,209
105	42,012	41,474	40,955	40,452	39,966	39,495	39,038
110	40,886	40,359	39,850	39,358	38,882	38,421	37,974
115	39,857	39,341	38,842	38,359	37,892	37,440	37,002
120	38,915	38,408	37,918	37,444	36,985	36,541	36,111
125	38,047	37,549	37,067	36,601	36,150	35,714	35,291
130	37,247	36,756	36,282	35,824	35,380	34,950	34,534
135	36,505	36,022	35,555	35,104	34,667	34,244	33,834
140	35,817	35,341	34,881	34,435	34,004	33,587	33,183
145	35,176	34,706	34,252	33,813	33,388	32,976	32,577
150	34,578	34,114	33,666	33,232	32,812	32,406	32,012
155	34,019	33,560	33,117	32,688	32,274	31,872	31,483
160	33,494	33,041	32,603	32,179	31,769	31,372	30,987
165	33,001	32,553	32,120	31,700	31,295	30,902	30,521
170	32,537	32,094	31,665	31,250	30,848	30,460	30,083
175	32,100	31,661	31,236	30,825	30,428	30,043	29,670
180	31,687	31,252	30,831	30,424	30,030	29,649	29,279
185	31,296	30,865	30,448	30,045	29,654	29,276	28,910
190	30,926	30,499	30,085	29,685	29,298	28,923	28,560
195	30,575	30,151	29,741	29,344	28,960	28,589	28,228
200	30,242	29,821	29,414	29,020	28,639	28,270	27,913
205	29,924	29,507	29,103	28,712	28,334	27,968	27,613
210	29,622	29,207	28,806	28,418	28,043	27,680	27,328
215	29,334	28,922	28,524	28,139	27,766	27,405	27,055
220	29,059	28,650	28,254	27,872	27,501	27,143	26,795
225	28,796	28,390	27,996	27,616	27,248	26,892	26,547
230	28,545	28,141	27,750	27,372	27,006	26,652	26,309
235	28,304	27,902	27,514	27,138	26,775	26,423	26,082
240	28,073	27,674	27,288	26,914	26,553	26,203	25,864
245	27,852	27,455	27,071	26,699	26,340	25,992	25,655
250	27,640	27,245	26,863	26,493	26,136	25,789	25,454
255	27,436	27,043	26,663	26,295	25,939	25,595	25,261
260	27,240	26,848	26,470	26,104	25,750	25,408	25,076
265	27,051	26,661	26,285	25,921	25,569	25,228	24,897
270	26,869	26,481	26,107	25,744	25,394	25,054	24,725
275	26,694	26,308	25,935	25,574	25,225	24,887	24,560
280	26,525	26,141	25,769	25,410	25,063	24,726	24,400
285	26,362	25,979	25,609	25,252	24,906	24,571	24,246
290	26,204	25,823	25,455	25,099	24,754	24,420	24,097
295	26,052	25,673	25,306	24,951	24,608	24,275	23,953
300	25,905	25,527	25,162	24,808	24,466	24,135	23,814

ENERGY EXPENDITURE IN BODYSTEPS
Women Ages 56–60

5'5"	5'6"	5'7"	5'8"	5'9"	5'10"	5'11"	6'0"
39,757	39,318	38,893	38,480	38,079	37,689	37,311	36,943
38,596	38,167	37,751	37,347	36,955	36,574	36,204	35,844
37,541	37,121	36,713	36,318	35,934	35,561	35,199	34,846
36,577	36,165	35,766	35,378	35,001	34,636	34,280	33,935
35,694	35,289	34,897	34,516	34,147	33,787	33,438	33,099
34,881	34,484	34,098	33,724	33,360	33,007	32,664	32,330
34,131	33,740	33,360	32,992	32,634	32,287	31,949	31,621
33,436	33,051	32,677	32,314	31,962	31,620	31,287	30,964
32,791	32,411	32,043	31,685	31,338	31,000	30,673	30,354
32,191	31,816	31,452	31,099	30,757	30,424	30,100	29,786
31,630	31,260	30,901	30,553	30,214	29,886	29,566	29,256
31,106	30,740	30,386	30,041	29,707	29,382	29,067	28,760
30,614	30,253	29,902	29,562	29,231	28,910	28,598	28,295
30,153	29,795	29,448	29,111	28,784	28,467	28,158	27,858
29,718	29,364	29,021	28,687	28,364	28,049	27,744	27,447
29,308	28,958	28,618	28,288	27,967	27,656	27,353	27,059
28,921	28,574	28,237	27,910	27,593	27,284	26,985	26,693
28,555	28,211	27,877	27,553	27,239	26,933	26,636	26,347
28,208	27,867	27,536	27,215	26,903	26,600	26,305	26,019
27,879	27,541	27,213	26,894	26,585	26,284	25,992	25,708
27,567	27,231	26,905	26,589	26,282	25,984	25,694	25,412
27,270	26,936	26,613	26,299	25,994	25,698	25,411	25,131
26,986	26,655	26,334	26,023	25,720	25,426	25,141	24,863
26,716	26,388	26,069	25,759	25,459	25,167	24,883	24,608
26,459	26,132	25,815	25,508	25,210	24,920	24,638	24,364
26,212	25,888	25,573	25,268	24,971	24,683	24,403	24,131
25,977	25,654	25,342	25,038	24,743	24,457	24,179	23,908
25,751	25,431	25,120	24,818	24,525	24,240	23,964	23,695
25,535	25,216	24,907	24,607	24,316	24,033	23,758	23,490
25,328	25,011	24,703	24,405	24,115	23,834	23,560	23,294
25,129	24,814	24,508	24,211	23,923	23,643	23,371	23,106
24,938	24,624	24,320	24,024	23,738	23,459	23,188	22,925
24,754	24,442	24,139	23,845	23,560	23,283	23,013	22,751
24,577	24,266	23,965	23,672	23,388	23,113	22,845	22,584
24,406	24,097	23,797	23,506	23,224	22,949	22,682	22,423
24,242	23,934	23,636	23,346	23,065	22,791	22,526	22,267
24,084	23,778	23,480	23,192	22,912	22,639	22,375	22,118
23,931	23,626	23,330	23,043	22,764	22,493	22,229	21,973
23,784	23,480	23,185	22,899	22,621	22,351	22,089	21,834
23,641	23,339	23,045	22,760	22,483	22,214	21,953	21,699
23,503	23,202	22,909	22,625	22,350	22,082	21,822	21,569

ENERGY EXPENDITURE IN BODYSTEPS
Women Ages 61–65

Weight	Height 4'10"	4'11"	5'0"	5'1"	5'2"	5'3"	5'4"
100	42,323	41,789	41,272	40,773	40,290	39,822	39,368
105	41,128	40,606	40,100	39,612	39,139	38,681	38,237
110	40,042	39,530	39,035	38,556	38,093	37,644	37,209
115	39,050	38,548	38,062	37,592	37,137	36,697	36,270
120	38,141	37,647	37,170	36,708	36,262	35,829	35,410
125	37,305	36,819	36,350	35,895	35,456	35,030	34,618
130	36,533	36,055	35,592	35,145	34,712	34,293	33,887
135	35,818	35,347	34,891	34,450	34,024	33,611	33,211
140	35,154	34,689	34,240	33,805	33,384	32,977	32,582
145	34,536	34,077	33,634	33,204	32,789	32,387	31,997
150	33,959	33,506	33,068	32,644	32,233	31,836	31,451
155	33,420	32,972	32,538	32,119	31,714	31,321	30,940
160	32,914	32,471	32,042	31,628	31,226	30,838	30,462
165	32,439	32,000	31,576	31,166	30,769	30,384	30,012
170	31,992	31,557	31,137	30,731	30,338	29,957	29,588
175	31,570	31,139	30,723	30,321	29,932	29,555	29,189
180	31,172	30,745	30,333	29,934	29,548	29,174	28,812
185	30,795	30,372	29,963	29,568	29,185	28,815	28,456
190	30,438	30,019	29,613	29,221	28,841	28,474	28,118
195	30,099	29,683	29,281	28,892	28,515	28,150	27,797
200	29,778	29,365	28,965	28,579	28,205	27,843	27,493
205	29,472	29,062	28,665	28,282	27,910	27,551	27,203
210	29,180	28,773	28,379	27,998	27,630	27,273	26,927
215	28,902	28,498	28,107	27,728	27,362	27,008	26,664
220	28,637	28,235	27,846	27,470	27,107	26,754	26,413
225	28,384	27,984	27,598	27,224	26,862	26,512	26,173
230	28,141	27,744	27,360	26,988	26,629	26,281	25,944
235	27,909	27,514	27,132	26,763	26,405	26,059	25,724
240	27,687	27,294	26,914	26,547	26,191	25,847	25,513
245	27,473	27,083	26,705	26,339	25,986	25,643	25,311
250	27,269	26,880	26,504	26,140	25,788	25,448	25,118
255	27,072	26,685	26,311	25,949	25,599	25,260	24,931
260	26,883	26,497	26,125	25,765	25,416	25,079	24,752
265	26,701	26,317	25,946	25,588	25,241	24,905	24,580
270	26,525	26,143	25,774	25,418	25,072	24,738	24,414
275	26,356	25,976	25,609	25,253	24,909	24,576	24,254
280	26,193	25,815	25,449	25,095	24,752	24,421	24,100
285	26,036	25,659	25,295	24,942	24,601	24,271	23,951
290	25,884	25,509	25,146	24,795	24,455	24,126	23,807
295	25,738	25,364	25,002	24,652	24,314	23,986	23,668
300	25,596	25,223	24,863	24,514	24,177	23,850	23,534

ENERGY EXPENDITURE IN BODYSTEPS
Women Ages 61–65

5'5"	5'6"	5'7"	5'8"	5'9"	5'10"	5'11"	6'0"
38,929	38,503	38,090	37,688	37,299	36,920	36,553	36,195
37,808	37,391	36,986	36,594	36,213	35,842	35,482	35,133
36,788	36,379	35,983	35,598	35,225	34,862	34,509	34,167
35,857	35,456	35,067	34,690	34,323	33,967	33,621	33,285
35,004	34,610	34,228	33,857	33,497	33,147	32,807	32,476
34,219	33,831	33,455	33,090	32,736	32,392	32,058	31,732
33,494	33,112	32,742	32,383	32,034	31,695	31,366	31,046
32,823	32,447	32,082	31,728	31,384	31,050	30,726	30,410
32,200	31,829	31,469	31,120	30,781	30,451	30,131	29,820
31,620	31,254	30,898	30,554	30,219	29,894	29,578	29,270
31,078	30,717	30,366	30,025	29,694	29,373	29,061	28,757
30,572	30,214	29,867	29,531	29,204	28,886	28,577	28,277
30,097	29,743	29,400	29,067	28,744	28,430	28,124	27,828
29,651	29,301	28,961	28,632	28,312	28,001	27,699	27,405
29,231	28,884	28,548	28,222	27,905	27,597	27,298	27,007
28,835	28,492	28,159	27,835	27,522	27,217	26,920	26,632
28,461	28,121	27,791	27,471	27,159	26,857	26,564	26,278
28,108	27,770	27,443	27,125	26,817	26,517	26,226	25,943
27,773	27,438	27,113	26,798	26,492	26,195	25,906	25,626
27,455	27,123	26,801	26,488	26,185	25,890	25,603	25,324
27,153	26,823	26,504	26,193	25,892	25,599	25,315	25,038
26,866	26,538	26,221	25,913	25,614	25,323	25,041	24,766
26,592	26,267	25,952	25,646	25,349	25,060	24,780	24,507
26,331	26,008	25,695	25,391	25,096	24,810	24,531	24,260
26,082	25,762	25,450	25,148	24,855	24,570	24,293	24,024
25,844	25,526	25,216	24,916	24,625	24,341	24,066	23,799
25,617	25,300	24,992	24,694	24,404	24,123	23,849	23,583
25,399	25,084	24,778	24,481	24,193	23,913	23,641	23,377
25,190	24,877	24,573	24,277	23,991	23,713	23,442	23,179
24,990	24,678	24,376	24,082	23,797	23,520	23,251	22,989
24,798	24,487	24,186	23,894	23,611	23,335	23,067	22,807
24,613	24,304	24,005	23,714	23,432	23,158	22,891	22,632
24,435	24,128	23,830	23,541	23,260	22,987	22,722	22,464
24,264	23,958	23,662	23,374	23,094	22,822	22,558	22,302
24,100	23,795	23,500	23,213	22,935	22,664	22,401	22,146
23,941	23,638	23,344	23,058	22,781	22,512	22,250	21,996
23,788	23,486	23,193	22,909	22,633	22,365	22,104	21,851
23,641	23,340	23,048	22,765	22,490	22,223	21,963	21,711
23,498	23,199	22,908	22,626	22,352	22,086	21,827	21,576
23,361	23,062	22,773	22,492	22,219	21,954	21,696	21,446
23,227	22,930	22,642	22,362	22,090	21,826	21,569	21,319

ENERGY EXPENDITURE IN BODYSTEPS
Women Ages 66–70

Weight	Height 4'10"	4'11"	5'0"	5'1"	5'2"	5'3"	5'4"
100	41,395	40,877	40,375	39,891	39,422	38,967	38,528
105	40,244	39,737	39,246	38,771	38,312	37,867	37,437
110	39,198	38,701	38,219	37,754	37,303	36,867	36,445
115	38,243	37,754	37,282	36,825	36,382	35,954	35,539
120	37,368	36,887	36,423	35,973	35,538	35,117	34,709
125	36,563	36,089	35,632	35,190	34,761	34,347	33,945
130	35,819	35,353	34,902	34,466	34,045	33,636	33,240
135	35,131	34,671	34,227	33,797	33,381	32,978	32,588
140	34,491	34,038	33,599	33,175	32,764	32,367	31,982
145	33,896	33,448	33,015	32,596	32,190	31,798	31,417
150	33,341	32,898	32,470	32,055	31,655	31,267	30,891
155	32,821	32,383	31,960	31,550	31,154	30,770	30,398
160	32,334	31,901	31,481	31,076	30,684	30,304	29,936
165	31,876	31,447	31,032	30,631	30,242	29,866	29,502
170	31,446	31,021	30,609	30,212	29,827	29,455	29,094
175	31,040	30,618	30,211	29,817	29,436	29,066	28,709
180	30,656	30,238	29,834	29,444	29,066	28,700	28,345
185	30,293	29,879	29,478	29,091	28,716	28,353	28,001
190	29,950	29,538	29,141	28,756	28,384	28,024	27,675
195	29,624	29,215	28,821	28,439	28,070	27,712	27,366
200	29,314	28,908	28,517	28,138	27,771	27,416	27,072
205	29,019	28,617	28,228	27,851	27,487	27,134	26,793
210	28,738	28,339	27,952	27,578	27,216	26,866	26,527
215	28,471	28,073	27,689	27,318	26,958	26,610	26,273
220	28,215	27,820	27,439	27,069	26,712	26,366	26,031
225	27,971	27,579	27,199	26,832	26,477	26,133	25,799
230	27,738	27,347	26,970	26,605	26,252	25,909	25,578
235	27,514	27,126	26,751	26,387	26,036	25,696	25,366
240	27,300	26,914	26,540	26,179	25,829	25,491	25,163
245	27,095	26,710	26,339	25,979	25,631	25,294	24,968
250	26,897	26,515	26,145	25,787	25,441	25,106	24,781
255	26,708	26,327	25,959	25,603	25,258	24,925	24,601
260	26,526	26,147	25,780	25,426	25,083	24,750	24,429
265	26,350	25,973	25,608	25,255	24,913	24,583	24,262
270	26,182	25,806	25,442	25,091	24,751	24,421	24,102
275	26,019	25,644	25,283	24,933	24,594	24,266	23,948
280	25,862	25,489	25,129	24,780	24,442	24,116	23,799
285	25,711	25,339	24,980	24,633	24,296	23,971	23,656
290	25,564	25,194	24,836	24,490	24,155	23,831	23,517
295	25,423	25,054	24,698	24,353	24,019	23,696	23,383
300	25,287	24,919	24,564	24,220	23,888	23,566	23,254

ENERGY EXPENDITURE IN BODYSTEPS
Women Ages 66–70

5'5"	5'6"	5'7"	5'8"	5'9"	5'10"	5'11"	6'0"
38,101	37,688	37,286	36,897	36,519	36,152	35,795	35,448
37,019	36,614	36,221	35,840	35,470	35,110	34,760	34,421
36,035	35,638	35,253	34,879	34,516	34,163	33,820	33,487
35,137	34,747	34,369	34,001	33,645	33,299	32,962	32,635
34,314	33,930	33,558	33,197	32,847	32,506	32,175	31,853
33,556	33,179	32,813	32,457	32,112	31,777	31,451	31,134
32,857	32,485	32,124	31,774	31,434	31,104	30,783	30,471
32,210	31,843	31,487	31,142	30,806	30,481	30,164	29,856
31,608	31,246	30,895	30,554	30,224	29,902	29,590	29,286
31,049	30,691	30,344	30,008	29,681	29,363	29,055	28,755
30,526	30,173	29,830	29,497	29,174	28,860	28,555	28,259
30,038	29,688	29,349	29,020	28,700	28,390	28,088	27,795
29,579	29,234	28,898	28,572	28,256	27,949	27,651	27,360
29,149	28,807	28,474	28,152	27,839	27,535	27,239	26,952
28,744	28,405	28,076	27,756	27,446	27,145	26,852	26,567
28,362	28,026	27,700	27,383	27,076	26,777	26,487	26,205
28,001	27,668	27,345	27,031	26,726	26,430	26,142	25,863
27,660	27,330	27,009	26,698	26,395	26,102	25,816	25,539
27,337	27,009	26,691	26,382	26,082	25,791	25,507	25,232
27,030	26,705	26,389	26,082	25,785	25,495	25,214	24,941
26,739	26,416	26,102	25,798	25,502	25,215	24,936	24,665
26,462	26,141	25,829	25,527	25,233	24,948	24,671	24,402
26,198	25,879	25,569	25,269	24,977	24,694	24,419	24,151
25,946	25,629	25,322	25,023	24,733	24,452	24,178	23,912
25,706	25,391	25,085	24,789	24,501	24,221	23,949	23,684
25,476	25,163	24,859	24,564	24,278	24,000	23,729	23,467
25,257	24,945	24,643	24,350	24,065	23,788	23,520	23,258
25,047	24,737	24,436	24,145	23,861	23,586	23,319	23,059
24,845	24,537	24,238	23,948	23,666	23,392	23,126	22,867
24,652	24,345	24,048	23,759	23,479	23,206	22,941	22,684
24,466	24,161	23,865	23,578	23,299	23,028	22,764	22,508
24,288	23,984	23,690	23,404	23,126	22,856	22,594	22,339
24,117	23,814	23,521	23,236	22,960	22,691	22,430	22,176
23,952	23,651	23,359	23,075	22,800	22,532	22,272	22,020
23,793	23,493	23,202	22,920	22,646	22,380	22,121	21,869
23,640	23,341	23,052	22,771	22,497	22,232	21,974	21,724
23,492	23,195	22,906	22,626	22,354	22,090	21,833	21,584
23,350	23,054	22,766	22,487	22,216	21,953	21,697	21,449
23,213	22,917	22,631	22,353	22,083	21,821	21,566	21,318
23,080	22,786	22,500	22,223	21,954	21,693	21,439	21,192
22,951	22,658	22,374	22,098	21,830	21,569	21,316	21,070

ENERGY EXPENDITURE IN BODYSTEPS
Women Ages 71–75

Weight	Height 4'10"	4'11"	5'0"	5'1"	5'2"	5'3"	5'4"
100	40,467	39,964	39,339	38,871	38,418	37,980	37,555
105	39,361	38,868	38,259	37,800	37,356	36,927	36,511
110	38,355	37,871	37,277	36,827	36,391	35,969	35,561
115	37,436	36,961	36,380	35,938	35,510	35,095	34,694
120	36,595	36,127	35,558	35,123	34,702	34,294	33,899
125	35,820	35,360	34,802	34,374	33,959	33,557	33,168
130	35,105	34,651	34,105	33,682	33,273	32,876	32,493
135	34,443	33,995	33,458	33,041	32,637	32,246	31,868
140	33,829	33,386	32,858	32,446	32,047	31,661	31,287
145	33,256	32,819	32,300	31,892	31,498	31,117	30,747
150	32,722	32,290	31,778	31,376	30,986	30,608	30,243
155	32,223	31,795	31,291	30,892	30,506	30,133	29,771
160	31,754	31,330	30,833	30,439	30,057	29,687	29,328
165	31,314	30,894	30,404	30,013	29,634	29,268	28,913
170	30,900	30,484	29,999	29,612	29,237	28,874	28,522
175	30,509	30,097	29,618	29,234	28,862	28,502	28,153
180	30,141	29,731	29,258	28,877	28,508	28,151	27,805
185	29,792	29,386	28,918	28,539	28,173	27,819	27,476
190	29,461	29,058	28,595	28,220	27,856	27,504	27,163
195	29,148	28,748	28,289	27,916	27,555	27,206	26,867
200	28,850	28,452	27,998	27,628	27,269	26,922	26,586
205	28,566	28,172	27,722	27,354	26,998	26,653	26,319
210	28,297	27,904	27,458	27,092	26,739	26,396	26,064
215	28,039	27,649	27,207	26,843	26,492	26,151	25,821
220	27,794	27,406	26,967	26,606	26,256	25,917	25,589
225	27,559	27,173	26,738	26,379	26,031	25,694	25,367
230	27,334	26,951	26,519	26,161	25,815	25,480	25,155
235	27,120	26,738	26,309	25,953	25,609	25,275	24,952
240	26,914	26,534	26,108	25,754	25,411	25,079	24,758
245	26,716	26,338	25,915	25,563	25,222	24,891	24,571
250	26,526	26,150	25,730	25,379	25,040	24,711	24,392
255	26,344	25,969	25,552	25,203	24,865	24,537	24,220
260	26,169	25,796	25,381	25,033	24,697	24,371	24,055
265	26,000	25,629	25,217	24,870	24,535	24,210	23,896
270	25,838	25,468	25,058	24,713	24,379	24,056	23,742
275	25,681	25,313	24,905	24,562	24,229	23,907	23,595
280	25,531	25,163	24,758	24,416	24,084	23,763	23,452
285	25,385	25,019	24,616	24,275	23,944	23,624	23,315
290	25,244	24,880	24,479	24,139	23,809	23,491	23,182
295	25,109	24,745	24,346	24,007	23,679	23,361	23,054
300	24,977	24,615	24,218	23,880	23,553	23,236	22,930

ENERGY EXPENDITURE IN BODYSTEPS
Women Ages 71–75

5'5"	5'6"	5'7"	5'8"	5'9"	5'10"	5'11"	6'0"
37,144	36,745	36,358	35,982	35,617	35,263	34,918	34,583
36,107	35,716	35,337	34,968	34,611	34,263	33,926	33,598
35,165	34,781	34,409	34,047	33,696	33,355	33,024	32,701
34,305	33,927	33,561	33,206	32,861	32,526	32,200	31,883
33,516	33,145	32,784	32,435	32,095	31,765	31,445	31,133
32,790	32,425	32,070	31,725	31,391	31,066	30,750	30,443
32,121	31,760	31,410	31,070	30,741	30,420	30,109	29,806
31,501	31,145	30,799	30,464	30,139	29,822	29,515	29,216
30,925	30,573	30,232	29,901	29,579	29,267	28,964	28,669
30,389	30,041	29,704	29,377	29,059	28,750	28,450	28,159
29,888	29,544	29,211	28,887	28,573	28,268	27,971	27,683
29,420	29,080	28,750	28,430	28,119	27,817	27,523	27,238
28,981	28,644	28,318	28,001	27,693	27,394	27,103	26,820
28,569	28,235	27,912	27,597	27,292	26,996	26,708	26,428
28,181	27,850	27,529	27,218	26,916	26,622	26,337	26,059
27,815	27,487	27,169	26,860	26,561	26,269	25,986	25,711
27,470	27,144	26,829	26,523	26,225	25,936	25,656	25,383
27,143	26,820	26,507	26,203	25,908	25,621	25,343	25,072
26,833	26,513	26,202	25,900	25,607	25,323	25,046	24,777
26,539	26,221	25,913	25,613	25,322	25,040	24,765	24,498
26,260	25,944	25,638	25,340	25,051	24,771	24,498	24,233
25,995	25,681	25,376	25,081	24,793	24,515	24,244	23,980
25,742	25,430	25,127	24,833	24,548	24,271	24,002	23,740
25,501	25,191	24,890	24,598	24,314	24,039	23,771	23,510
25,271	24,962	24,663	24,373	24,091	23,817	23,550	23,292
25,051	24,744	24,447	24,158	23,877	23,605	23,340	23,082
24,841	24,535	24,239	23,952	23,673	23,402	23,139	22,882
24,639	24,336	24,041	23,755	23,478	23,208	22,946	22,691
24,446	24,144	23,851	23,566	23,290	23,022	22,761	22,507
24,261	23,960	23,669	23,385	23,111	22,843	22,584	22,331
24,084	23,784	23,494	23,212	22,938	22,672	22,414	22,162
23,913	23,615	23,326	23,045	22,772	22,507	22,250	22,000
23,749	23,452	23,164	22,884	22,613	22,349	22,093	21,844
23,591	23,295	23,008	22,730	22,460	22,197	21,942	21,694
23,439	23,144	22,858	22,581	22,312	22,050	21,796	21,549
23,292	22,999	22,714	22,438	22,170	21,909	21,656	21,410
23,151	22,858	22,575	22,300	22,032	21,773	21,520	21,275
23,014	22,723	22,440	22,166	21,900	21,641	21,390	21,145
22,883	22,592	22,311	22,037	21,772	21,514	21,264	21,020
22,755	22,466	22,185	21,913	21,649	21,392	21,142	20,899
22,632	22,344	22,064	21,793	21,529	21,273	21,024	20,782

ENERGY EXPENDITURE IN BODYSTEPS
Women Ages 76–80

Weight	Height 4'10"	4'11"	5'0"	5'1"	5'2"	5'3"	5'4"
100	39,539	39,052	38,282	37,832	37,396	36,974	36,565
105	38,477	37,999	37,253	36,811	36,383	35,969	35,568
110	37,511	37,042	36,317	35,882	35,462	35,055	34,661
115	36,630	36,168	35,462	35,035	34,621	34,221	33,833
120	35,821	35,367	34,678	34,258	33,850	33,456	33,074
125	35,078	34,630	33,958	33,543	33,141	32,752	32,376
130	34,391	33,949	33,292	32,883	32,486	32,103	31,731
135	33,756	33,319	32,676	32,272	31,880	31,501	31,134
140	33,166	32,735	32,104	31,704	31,317	30,943	30,580
145	32,616	32,190	31,571	31,176	30,793	30,423	30,064
150	32,104	31,682	31,074	30,683	30,304	29,938	29,582
155	31,624	31,206	30,609	30,222	29,847	29,484	29,132
160	31,174	30,760	30,173	29,789	29,418	29,058	28,710
165	30,752	30,341	29,764	29,383	29,015	28,658	28,313
170	30,354	29,947	29,378	29,001	28,636	28,282	27,939
175	29,979	29,576	29,015	28,640	28,278	27,927	27,587
180	29,625	29,225	28,672	28,300	27,940	27,592	27,255
185	29,290	28,893	28,347	27,978	27,621	27,275	26,940
190	28,973	28,578	28,039	27,673	27,318	26,975	26,642
195	28,672	28,280	27,747	27,383	27,031	26,690	26,360
200	28,386	27,996	27,470	27,108	26,758	26,419	26,091
205	28,114	27,727	27,207	26,847	26,499	26,162	25,836
210	27,855	27,470	26,955	26,598	26,252	25,917	25,592
215	27,608	27,225	26,716	26,360	26,016	25,683	25,360
220	27,372	26,991	26,487	26,134	25,791	25,460	25,139
225	27,147	26,768	26,269	25,917	25,576	25,247	24,927
230	26,931	26,554	26,060	25,710	25,371	25,043	24,725
235	26,725	26,350	25,860	25,511	25,174	24,847	24,531
240	26,527	26,154	25,668	25,321	24,985	24,660	24,345
245	26,337	25,966	25,484	25,139	24,805	24,481	24,167
250	26,155	25,785	25,308	24,964	24,631	24,309	23,996
255	25,980	25,612	25,138	24,796	24,464	24,143	23,832
260	25,812	25,445	24,975	24,634	24,304	23,984	23,674
265	25,650	25,284	24,818	24,478	24,149	23,831	23,522
270	25,494	25,130	24,667	24,328	24,000	23,683	23,376
275	25,344	24,981	24,521	24,184	23,857	23,541	23,234
280	25,199	24,837	24,381	24,045	23,719	23,404	23,098
285	25,059	24,699	24,246	23,910	23,586	23,272	22,967
290	24,924	24,565	24,115	23,780	23,457	23,144	22,840
295	24,794	24,436	23,988	23,655	23,333	23,020	22,718
300	24,668	24,311	23,866	23,534	23,212	22,901	22,600

ENERGY EXPENDITURE IN BODYSTEPS
Women Ages 76–80

5'5"	5'6"	5'7"	5'8"	5'9"	5'10"	5'11"	6'0"
36,169	35,785	35,412	35,050	34,699	34,357	34,026	33,703
35,179	34,802	34,436	34,081	33,736	33,401	33,076	32,759
34,279	33,908	33,549	33,200	32,861	32,532	32,212	31,901
33,457	33,092	32,739	32,396	32,062	31,738	31,424	31,118
32,704	32,345	31,996	31,658	31,330	31,011	30,701	30,400
32,011	31,657	31,313	30,980	30,656	30,342	30,036	29,739
31,371	31,021	30,682	30,354	30,034	29,724	29,422	29,129
30,778	30,433	30,099	29,774	29,458	29,152	28,854	28,564
30,228	29,887	29,556	29,235	28,923	28,621	28,326	28,040
29,716	29,379	29,052	28,734	28,426	28,126	27,835	27,552
29,238	28,904	28,581	28,266	27,961	27,664	27,376	27,096
28,791	28,460	28,140	27,828	27,526	27,233	26,947	26,670
28,372	28,044	27,727	27,418	27,119	26,828	26,545	26,270
27,978	27,653	27,338	27,033	26,736	26,448	26,167	25,895
27,607	27,285	26,973	26,670	26,376	26,090	25,812	25,541
27,258	26,939	26,629	26,328	26,036	25,752	25,476	25,208
26,928	26,611	26,303	26,005	25,715	25,433	25,160	24,894
26,616	26,301	25,996	25,699	25,411	25,132	24,860	24,596
26,320	26,007	25,704	25,410	25,124	24,846	24,576	24,314
26,039	25,729	25,428	25,135	24,851	24,575	24,307	24,047
25,773	25,464	25,165	24,874	24,592	24,318	24,052	23,793
25,519	25,212	24,915	24,626	24,346	24,073	23,808	23,551
25,278	24,973	24,677	24,390	24,111	23,840	23,577	23,321
25,047	24,744	24,450	24,164	23,887	23,617	23,356	23,101
24,828	24,526	24,233	23,949	23,673	23,405	23,145	22,892
24,618	24,317	24,026	23,744	23,469	23,202	22,943	22,691
24,417	24,118	23,828	23,547	23,274	23,008	22,751	22,500
24,224	23,927	23,639	23,359	23,087	22,823	22,566	22,316
24,040	23,744	23,457	23,178	22,908	22,645	22,389	22,141
23,863	23,569	23,283	23,005	22,736	22,474	22,219	21,972
23,694	23,400	23,115	22,839	22,571	22,310	22,057	21,810
23,531	23,238	22,955	22,679	22,412	22,152	21,900	21,655
23,374	23,083	22,800	22,526	22,260	22,001	21,750	21,505
23,223	22,933	22,651	22,378	22,113	21,855	21,605	21,362
23,078	22,788	22,508	22,236	21,972	21,715	21,466	21,223
22,937	22,650	22,370	22,099	21,836	21,580	21,331	21,090
22,802	22,515	22,237	21,967	21,704	21,449	21,202	20,961
22,672	22,386	22,109	21,839	21,578	21,324	21,077	20,837
22,546	22,261	21,985	21,716	21,455	21,202	20,956	20,717
22,425	22,141	21,865	21,597	21,337	21,085	20,839	20,601
22,307	22,024	21,749	21,482	21,223	20,971	20,727	20,489

ENERGY EXPENDITURE IN BODYSTEPS
Women Ages 81–85

Weight	Height 4'10"	4'11"	5'0"	5'1"	5'2"	5'3"	5'4"
100	38,611	38,140	37,207	36,774	36,356	35,950	35,557
105	37,593	37,130	36,229	35,803	35,392	34,994	34,608
110	36,668	36,213	35,339	34,921	34,516	34,124	33,744
115	35,823	35,375	34,527	34,115	33,716	33,330	32,956
120	35,048	34,607	33,782	33,376	32,983	32,602	32,234
125	34,335	33,900	33,097	32,696	32,309	31,933	31,569
130	33,678	33,248	32,465	32,069	31,686	31,315	30,956
135	33,069	32,644	31,880	31,488	31,109	30,743	30,387
140	32,503	32,083	31,336	30,949	30,574	30,211	29,860
145	31,976	31,561	30,830	30,447	30,076	29,717	29,369
150	31,485	31,073	30,357	29,978	29,611	29,255	28,910
155	31,025	30,618	29,916	29,539	29,175	28,823	28,482
160	30,594	30,190	29,501	29,128	28,767	28,418	28,080
165	30,189	29,789	29,112	28,742	28,384	28,038	27,702
170	29,808	29,411	28,746	28,379	28,024	27,680	27,346
175	29,449	29,054	28,400	28,036	27,683	27,342	27,011
180	29,110	28,718	28,074	27,712	27,362	27,023	26,695
185	28,789	28,400	27,766	27,406	27,058	26,722	26,395
190	28,484	28,098	27,473	27,116	26,771	26,436	26,112
195	28,196	27,812	27,196	26,841	26,498	26,165	25,843
200	27,922	27,540	26,933	26,580	26,238	25,907	25,587
205	27,661	27,282	26,682	26,331	25,991	25,662	25,344
210	27,413	27,035	26,443	26,094	25,756	25,429	25,112
215	27,176	26,801	26,216	25,868	25,532	25,207	24,891
220	26,950	26,577	25,999	25,653	25,318	24,994	24,681
225	26,734	26,362	25,791	25,447	25,114	24,792	24,479
230	26,528	26,158	25,592	25,250	24,918	24,597	24,287
235	26,330	25,961	25,402	25,061	24,731	24,412	24,102
240	26,140	25,774	25,220	24,881	24,552	24,234	23,925
245	25,958	25,593	25,045	24,707	24,380	24,063	23,756
250	25,784	25,420	24,878	24,541	24,215	23,899	23,593
255	25,616	25,254	24,716	24,381	24,056	23,741	23,437
260	25,455	25,094	24,562	24,227	23,903	23,590	23,286
265	25,300	24,940	24,412	24,079	23,756	23,444	23,142
270	25,150	24,792	24,269	23,937	23,615	23,304	23,002
275	25,007	24,649	24,130	23,799	23,479	23,169	22,868
280	24,868	24,512	23,997	23,667	23,347	23,038	22,738
285	24,734	24,379	23,868	23,539	23,221	22,912	22,613
290	24,604	24,251	23,744	23,416	23,098	22,791	22,493
295	24,479	24,127	23,624	23,297	22,980	22,673	22,376
300	24,359	24,007	23,508	23,181	22,866	22,560	22,264

ENERGY EXPENDITURE IN BODYSTEPS
Women Ages 81–85

5'5"	5'6"	5'7"	5'8"	5'9"	5'10"	5'11"	6'0"
35,176	34,807	34,449	34,101	33,764	33,436	33,117	32,807
34,234	33,871	33,519	33,177	32,846	32,524	32,210	31,906
33,376	33,020	32,673	32,337	32,011	31,694	31,386	31,087
32,594	32,242	31,901	31,571	31,249	30,937	30,634	30,339
31,876	31,530	31,194	30,868	30,551	30,243	29,944	29,653
31,216	30,875	30,543	30,221	29,908	29,604	29,309	29,022
30,607	30,269	29,942	29,624	29,315	29,015	28,723	28,440
30,043	29,709	29,385	29,071	28,766	28,469	28,181	27,901
29,519	29,189	28,869	28,558	28,256	27,962	27,677	27,400
29,032	28,705	28,388	28,080	27,781	27,490	27,208	26,934
28,577	28,253	27,939	27,634	27,338	27,050	26,770	26,499
28,151	27,830	27,519	27,216	26,923	26,638	26,361	26,092
27,752	27,433	27,125	26,825	26,534	26,252	25,977	25,710
27,377	27,061	26,755	26,458	26,169	25,889	25,617	25,352
27,024	26,710	26,407	26,112	25,826	25,547	25,277	25,014
26,691	26,380	26,078	25,786	25,502	25,225	24,957	24,696
26,377	26,068	25,768	25,478	25,196	24,921	24,655	24,396
26,079	25,773	25,475	25,186	24,906	24,634	24,369	24,112
25,798	25,493	25,197	24,910	24,632	24,361	24,098	23,843
25,530	25,228	24,934	24,649	24,372	24,103	23,841	23,587
25,277	24,975	24,683	24,400	24,125	23,857	23,597	23,344
25,035	24,736	24,445	24,163	23,889	23,623	23,365	23,114
24,805	24,507	24,218	23,938	23,665	23,401	23,144	22,894
24,586	24,289	24,002	23,723	23,452	23,189	22,933	22,684
24,377	24,082	23,796	23,518	23,248	22,986	22,732	22,484
24,177	23,883	23,598	23,322	23,053	22,793	22,539	22,293
23,985	23,693	23,410	23,134	22,867	22,608	22,355	22,110
23,802	23,511	23,229	22,955	22,689	22,430	22,179	21,935
23,627	23,337	23,056	22,783	22,518	22,261	22,011	21,767
23,458	23,170	22,890	22,618	22,354	22,098	21,849	21,606
23,297	23,009	22,730	22,459	22,197	21,941	21,693	21,452
23,141	22,855	22,577	22,307	22,045	21,791	21,544	21,303
22,992	22,707	22,430	22,161	21,900	21,647	21,400	21,161
22,848	22,564	22,288	22,020	21,760	21,508	21,262	21,023
22,710	22,426	22,151	21,885	21,625	21,374	21,129	20,891
22,577	22,294	22,020	21,754	21,496	21,245	21,001	20,764
22,448	22,166	21,893	21,628	21,370	21,120	20,877	20,641
22,324	22,043	21,771	21,506	21,250	21,000	20,758	20,522
22,204	21,924	21,653	21,389	21,133	20,884	20,643	20,408
22,088	21,809	21,538	21,276	21,020	20,772	20,531	20,297
21,977	21,698	21,428	21,166	20,911	20,664	20,424	20,190

ENERGY EXPENDITURE IN BODYSTEPS
Women Ages 86–90

Weight	Height 4'10"	4'11"	5'0"	5'1"	5'2"	5'3"	5'4"
100	37,683	37,228	36,281	35,698	35,296	34,908	34,531
105	36,709	36,262	35,347	34,778	34,383	34,001	33,630
110	35,824	35,383	34,497	33,942	33,553	33,177	32,812
115	35,016	34,582	33,722	33,179	32,795	32,424	32,064
120	34,275	33,846	33,011	32,479	32,100	31,734	31,379
125	33,593	33,170	32,357	31,835	31,461	31,099	30,748
130	32,964	32,546	31,753	31,241	30,871	30,513	30,166
135	32,381	31,968	31,194	30,691	30,325	29,971	29,627
140	31,840	31,431	30,675	30,180	29,818	29,467	29,127
145	31,336	30,932	30,191	29,704	29,345	28,998	28,661
150	30,866	30,465	29,740	29,260	28,904	28,560	28,226
155	30,426	30,029	29,318	28,845	28,492	28,151	27,820
160	30,014	29,620	28,923	28,456	28,106	27,767	27,438
165	29,627	29,236	28,551	28,090	27,742	27,406	27,080
170	29,262	28,874	28,201	27,745	27,401	27,067	26,743
175	28,919	28,533	27,871	27,421	27,078	26,746	26,425
180	28,594	28,211	27,560	27,114	26,774	26,444	26,125
185	28,287	27,906	27,265	26,824	26,486	26,158	25,841
190	27,996	27,618	26,986	26,550	26,213	25,887	25,572
195	27,720	27,344	26,721	26,289	25,954	25,630	25,317
200	27,458	27,084	26,470	26,041	25,709	25,386	25,074
205	27,208	26,837	26,230	25,806	25,475	25,154	24,843
210	26,971	26,601	26,002	25,582	25,252	24,933	24,624
215	26,744	26,376	25,785	25,368	25,040	24,722	24,414
220	26,528	26,162	25,578	25,164	24,837	24,521	24,214
225	26,322	25,957	25,380	24,968	24,643	24,328	24,023
230	26,124	25,761	25,190	24,782	24,458	24,144	23,840
235	25,935	25,573	25,008	24,603	24,281	23,968	23,666
240	25,754	25,393	24,834	24,432	24,111	23,799	23,498
245	25,580	25,221	24,668	24,268	23,947	23,637	23,337
250	25,413	25,055	24,507	24,110	23,791	23,482	23,183
255	25,252	24,896	24,353	23,959	23,641	23,333	23,034
260	25,098	24,743	24,205	23,813	23,496	23,189	22,892
265	24,950	24,596	24,063	23,673	23,357	23,051	22,754
270	24,807	24,454	23,926	23,538	23,223	22,918	22,622
275	24,669	24,318	23,794	23,408	23,094	22,789	22,495
280	24,536	24,186	23,666	23,282	22,969	22,666	22,372
285	24,408	24,059	23,543	23,161	22,849	22,547	22,253
290	24,284	23,936	23,425	23,045	22,733	22,431	22,139
295	24,165	23,817	23,310	22,932	22,621	22,320	22,029
300	24,049	23,703	23,199	22,823	22,513	22,212	21,922

ENERGY EXPENDITURE IN BODYSTEPS
Women Ages 86–90

5'5"	5'6"	5'7"	5'8"	5'9"	5'10"	5'11"	6'0"
34,166	33,812	33,469	33,136	32,812	32,498	32,192	31,895
33,271	32,923	32,586	32,258	31,939	31,630	31,330	31,037
32,458	32,115	31,782	31,460	31,146	30,841	30,545	30,258
31,715	31,377	31,049	30,731	30,422	30,121	29,829	29,546
31,035	30,701	30,377	30,063	29,758	29,461	29,173	28,893
30,408	30,079	29,759	29,448	29,147	28,854	28,569	28,293
29,830	29,504	29,188	28,881	28,583	28,293	28,012	27,738
29,295	28,972	28,659	28,356	28,061	27,774	27,496	27,225
28,798	28,478	28,169	27,868	27,576	27,292	27,017	26,749
28,335	28,019	27,712	27,414	27,124	26,843	26,570	26,305
27,903	27,589	27,285	26,990	26,703	26,425	26,154	25,891
27,499	27,188	26,886	26,593	26,309	26,033	25,764	25,503
27,120	26,812	26,512	26,222	25,940	25,665	25,399	25,140
26,764	26,458	26,161	25,872	25,592	25,320	25,056	24,799
26,429	26,125	25,830	25,544	25,266	24,996	24,733	24,478
26,114	25,811	25,518	25,234	24,958	24,689	24,429	24,175
25,815	25,515	25,224	24,941	24,667	24,400	24,141	23,889
25,533	25,235	24,945	24,664	24,392	24,127	23,869	23,619
25,266	24,969	24,681	24,402	24,131	23,867	23,611	23,363
25,012	24,717	24,431	24,153	23,884	23,622	23,367	23,119
24,771	24,478	24,193	23,917	23,649	23,388	23,135	22,888
24,542	24,250	23,967	23,692	23,425	23,166	22,914	22,669
24,324	24,033	23,752	23,478	23,212	22,954	22,703	22,460
24,116	23,827	23,546	23,274	23,009	22,752	22,503	22,260
23,917	23,629	23,350	23,079	22,816	22,560	22,311	22,070
23,728	23,441	23,163	22,893	22,630	22,376	22,128	21,888
23,546	23,260	22,983	22,715	22,453	22,200	21,953	21,714
23,372	23,088	22,812	22,544	22,284	22,031	21,786	21,547
23,206	22,922	22,647	22,381	22,121	21,870	21,625	21,387
23,046	22,763	22,490	22,224	21,966	21,715	21,471	21,234
22,892	22,611	22,338	22,073	21,816	21,566	21,323	21,087
22,745	22,465	22,193	21,929	21,672	21,423	21,181	20,946
22,603	22,324	22,053	21,790	21,534	21,286	21,045	20,810
22,467	22,188	21,918	21,656	21,401	21,154	20,913	20,679
22,336	22,058	21,788	21,527	21,273	21,026	20,786	20,553
22,209	21,932	21,664	21,403	21,150	20,904	20,664	20,432
22,087	21,811	21,543	21,283	21,031	20,785	20,547	20,315
21,969	21,694	21,427	21,168	20,916	20,671	20,433	20,202
21,856	21,581	21,315	21,056	20,805	20,561	20,324	20,093
21,746	21,472	21,206	20,948	20,698	20,454	20,218	19,988
21,640	21,367	21,101	20,844	20,594	20,351	20,116	19,886

ENERGY EXPENDITURE IN BODYSTEPS
Men Ages 20–25

Weight	Height 5'2"	5'3"	5'4"	5'5"	5'6"	5'7"	5'8"
130	42,992	42,665	42,347	42,040	41,742	41,453	41,172
135	42,254	41,926	41,607	41,298	40,999	40,708	40,426
140	41,569	41,239	40,919	40,609	40,309	40,017	39,734
145	40,932	40,600	40,279	39,968	39,666	39,373	39,089
150	40,336	40,004	39,682	39,369	39,066	38,773	38,487
155	39,780	39,446	39,123	38,809	38,505	38,211	37,924
160	39,258	38,923	38,599	38,284	37,979	37,684	37,397
165	38,767	38,431	38,106	37,791	37,485	37,189	36,901
170	38,306	37,969	37,643	37,327	37,020	36,723	36,435
175	37,870	37,533	37,206	36,889	36,582	36,284	35,995
180	37,459	37,121	36,794	36,476	36,168	35,869	35,579
185	37,071	36,732	36,403	36,085	35,776	35,477	35,186
190	36,702	36,363	36,033	35,715	35,405	35,105	34,814
195	36,353	36,012	35,683	35,363	35,053	34,752	34,461
200	36,021	35,680	35,349	35,029	34,719	34,417	34,125
205	35,705	35,363	35,032	34,712	34,401	34,099	33,806
210	35,404	35,062	34,731	34,409	34,098	33,795	33,502
215	35,118	34,775	34,443	34,121	33,809	33,506	33,212
220	34,844	34,501	34,168	33,846	33,533	33,230	32,935
225	34,582	34,239	33,905	33,583	33,270	32,966	32,671
230	34,332	33,988	33,654	33,331	33,017	32,713	32,418
235	34,093	33,748	33,414	33,090	32,776	32,472	32,176
240	33,863	33,518	33,183	32,859	32,545	32,240	31,944
245	33,643	33,297	32,962	32,638	32,323	32,018	31,721
250	33,432	33,086	32,750	32,425	32,110	31,804	31,508
255	33,229	32,882	32,546	32,221	31,906	31,600	31,302
260	33,033	32,686	32,350	32,025	31,709	31,402	31,105
265	32,845	32,498	32,162	31,836	31,520	31,213	30,915
270	32,664	32,317	31,980	31,654	31,337	31,030	30,732
275	32,490	32,142	31,805	31,478	31,162	30,854	30,556
280	32,322	31,974	31,636	31,309	30,992	30,685	30,386
285	32,160	31,811	31,473	31,146	30,829	30,521	30,222
290	32,003	31,654	31,316	30,989	30,671	30,363	30,064
295	31,852	31,503	31,164	30,836	30,519	30,210	29,911
300	31,705	31,356	31,017	30,689	30,371	30,062	29,763
305	31,564	31,214	30,875	30,547	30,229	29,920	29,620
310	31,427	31,077	30,738	30,409	30,091	29,781	29,481

ENERGY EXPENDITURE IN BODYSTEPS
Men Ages 20–25

5'9"	5'10"	5'11"	6'0"	6'1"	6'2"	6'3"	6'4"	6'5"
40,899	40,634	40,377	40,127	39,883	39,647	39,416	39,192	38,973
40,152	39,886	39,628	39,377	39,132	38,894	38,663	38,437	38,218
39,459	39,192	38,932	38,680	38,434	38,196	37,963	37,737	37,516
38,813	38,545	38,284	38,031	37,785	37,545	37,312	37,085	36,863
38,210	37,941	37,680	37,426	37,179	36,938	36,704	36,476	36,254
37,647	37,377	37,114	36,859	36,611	36,370	36,135	35,907	35,684
37,118	36,847	36,584	36,329	36,080	35,838	35,602	35,373	35,149
36,622	36,350	36,086	35,830	35,580	35,338	35,101	34,871	34,647
36,154	35,882	35,618	35,360	35,110	34,867	34,630	34,399	34,175
35,714	35,441	35,176	34,918	34,667	34,423	34,186	33,954	33,729
35,298	35,024	34,758	34,500	34,248	34,004	33,766	33,534	33,308
34,904	34,630	34,363	34,104	33,852	33,607	33,369	33,136	32,910
34,531	34,256	33,989	33,730	33,477	33,232	32,993	32,760	32,533
34,177	33,902	33,634	33,374	33,121	32,875	32,636	32,402	32,175
33,841	33,565	33,297	33,037	32,783	32,537	32,297	32,063	31,835
33,521	33,245	32,977	32,716	32,462	32,215	31,974	31,740	31,512
33,217	32,940	32,671	32,410	32,155	31,908	31,667	31,433	31,204
32,927	32,649	32,380	32,118	31,863	31,615	31,374	31,139	30,911
32,650	32,372	32,102	31,840	31,585	31,336	31,095	30,859	30,630
32,385	32,107	31,836	31,574	31,318	31,070	30,828	30,592	30,362
32,131	31,853	31,582	31,319	31,063	30,814	30,572	30,336	30,106
31,889	31,610	31,339	31,076	30,819	30,570	30,327	30,091	29,861
31,657	31,377	31,106	30,842	30,586	30,336	30,093	29,856	29,626
31,434	31,154	30,882	30,618	30,361	30,111	29,868	29,631	29,401
31,220	30,940	30,668	30,403	30,146	29,896	29,652	29,415	29,184
31,014	30,734	30,462	30,197	29,939	29,689	29,445	29,207	28,976
30,816	30,536	30,263	29,998	29,740	29,490	29,245	29,008	28,776
30,626	30,345	30,072	29,807	29,549	29,298	29,054	28,816	28,584
30,443	30,162	29,889	29,623	29,365	29,113	28,869	28,631	28,399
30,266	29,985	29,712	29,446	29,187	28,936	28,691	28,452	28,220
30,096	29,814	29,541	29,275	29,016	28,764	28,519	28,280	28,048
29,932	29,650	29,376	29,110	28,851	28,599	28,353	28,114	27,882
29,773	29,491	29,217	28,950	28,691	28,439	28,193	27,954	27,721
29,620	29,338	29,063	28,796	28,537	28,285	28,039	27,800	27,566
29,472	29,189	28,915	28,648	28,388	28,135	27,889	27,650	27,417
29,329	29,046	28,771	28,504	28,244	27,991	27,745	27,505	27,272
29,190	28,907	28,632	28,365	28,104	27,851	27,605	27,365	27,132

ENERGY EXPENDITURE IN BODYSTEPS
Men Ages 26–30

Weight	Height						
	5'2"	5'3"	5'4"	5'5"	5'6"	5'7"	5'8"
130	41,933	41,622	41,322	41,030	40,747	40,473	40,206
135	41,235	40,922	40,619	40,325	40,041	39,764	39,496
140	40,586	40,271	39,967	39,671	39,385	39,107	38,837
145	39,982	39,666	39,359	39,062	38,774	38,495	38,223
150	39,419	39,101	38,792	38,494	38,204	37,923	37,651
155	38,891	38,572	38,262	37,962	37,671	37,389	37,115
160	38,397	38,076	37,765	37,463	37,171	36,888	36,612
165	37,933	37,610	37,298	36,995	36,702	36,417	36,140
170	37,496	37,172	36,858	36,554	36,260	35,974	35,696
175	37,084	36,759	36,444	36,139	35,843	35,556	35,277
180	36,695	36,368	36,053	35,746	35,449	35,161	34,882
185	36,326	35,999	35,682	35,375	35,077	34,788	34,508
190	35,978	35,650	35,332	35,023	34,725	34,435	34,153
195	35,647	35,318	34,999	34,690	34,390	34,099	33,817
200	35,333	35,002	34,683	34,373	34,072	33,781	33,497
205	35,034	34,703	34,382	34,071	33,770	33,477	33,194
210	34,749	34,417	34,096	33,784	33,482	33,189	32,904
215	34,477	34,145	33,822	33,510	33,207	32,913	32,628
220	34,218	33,885	33,562	33,249	32,945	32,651	32,365
225	33,971	33,636	33,313	32,999	32,695	32,400	32,113
230	33,734	33,399	33,074	32,760	32,455	32,159	31,872
235	33,507	33,171	32,846	32,531	32,226	31,930	31,642
240	33,290	32,953	32,628	32,312	32,006	31,709	31,421
245	33,081	32,744	32,418	32,102	31,795	31,498	31,209
250	32,881	32,544	32,217	31,900	31,593	31,295	31,006
255	32,689	32,351	32,023	31,706	31,398	31,100	30,810
260	32,504	32,165	31,837	31,520	31,211	30,912	30,622
265	32,326	31,987	31,658	31,340	31,032	30,732	30,441
270	32,155	31,815	31,486	31,167	30,858	30,558	30,267
275	31,989	31,649	31,320	31,001	30,691	30,391	30,100
280	31,830	31,490	31,160	30,840	30,530	30,230	29,938
285	31,677	31,336	31,005	30,685	30,375	30,074	29,782
290	31,528	31,187	30,856	30,536	30,225	29,924	29,631
295	31,385	31,043	30,712	30,391	30,080	29,778	29,485
300	31,246	30,904	30,573	30,252	29,940	29,638	29,344
305	31,113	30,770	30,438	30,116	29,805	29,502	29,208
310	30,983	30,640	30,308	29,986	29,673	29,371	29,077

APPENDIX B

ENERGY EXPENDITURE IN BODYSTEPS
Men Ages 26–30

5'9"	5'10"	5'11"	6'0"	6'1"	6'2"	6'3"	6'4"	6'5"
39,948	39,696	39,452	39,215	38,984	38,759	38,541	38,328	38,120
39,236	38,983	38,737	38,498	38,266	38,040	37,820	37,605	37,397
38,575	38,321	38,073	37,833	37,599	37,372	37,150	36,935	36,725
37,960	37,704	37,455	37,214	36,978	36,750	36,527	36,310	36,099
37,386	37,128	36,879	36,635	36,399	36,169	35,945	35,727	35,515
36,849	36,590	36,339	36,095	35,857	35,626	35,401	35,182	34,969
36,345	36,085	35,833	35,588	35,349	35,117	34,891	34,671	34,457
35,872	35,611	35,358	35,111	34,872	34,639	34,412	34,191	33,975
35,427	35,165	34,910	34,663	34,422	34,188	33,961	33,739	33,523
35,007	34,744	34,489	34,240	33,999	33,764	33,535	33,313	33,096
34,610	34,347	34,090	33,841	33,599	33,363	33,134	32,910	32,692
34,235	33,971	33,714	33,464	33,220	32,984	32,754	32,529	32,311
33,880	33,615	33,357	33,106	32,862	32,625	32,394	32,169	31,950
33,543	33,277	33,018	32,766	32,522	32,284	32,052	31,826	31,607
33,223	32,956	32,696	32,444	32,199	31,960	31,728	31,501	31,281
32,918	32,650	32,390	32,137	31,891	31,652	31,419	31,192	30,971
32,628	32,360	32,099	31,845	31,599	31,359	31,125	30,898	30,676
32,351	32,082	31,821	31,567	31,320	31,079	30,845	30,617	30,395
32,087	31,818	31,556	31,301	31,053	30,812	30,577	30,349	30,126
31,835	31,565	31,302	31,047	30,799	30,557	30,322	30,093	29,870
31,594	31,323	31,060	30,804	30,555	30,313	30,077	29,848	29,624
31,363	31,091	30,828	30,571	30,322	30,079	29,843	29,613	29,389
31,141	30,869	30,605	30,348	30,098	29,855	29,619	29,388	29,164
30,929	30,656	30,392	30,134	29,884	29,641	29,404	29,173	28,948
30,725	30,452	30,187	29,929	29,678	29,434	29,197	28,966	28,741
30,529	30,256	29,990	29,732	29,481	29,236	28,999	28,767	28,541
30,341	30,067	29,801	29,542	29,291	29,046	28,808	28,576	28,350
30,159	29,885	29,619	29,360	29,108	28,863	28,624	28,392	28,166
29,985	29,710	29,443	29,184	28,932	28,686	28,447	28,215	27,988
29,817	29,542	29,274	29,015	28,762	28,516	28,277	28,044	27,817
29,654	29,379	29,111	28,851	28,598	28,352	28,113	27,879	27,652
29,498	29,222	28,954	28,694	28,440	28,194	27,954	27,720	27,493
29,347	29,071	28,802	28,542	28,288	28,041	27,801	27,567	27,339
29,201	28,924	28,656	28,395	28,141	27,894	27,653	27,419	27,191
29,060	28,783	28,514	28,253	27,998	27,751	27,510	27,276	27,047
28,923	28,646	28,377	28,115	27,861	27,613	27,372	27,137	26,908
28,791	28,514	28,244	27,982	27,727	27,479	27,238	27,003	26,774

ENERGY EXPENDITURE IN BODYSTEPS
Men Ages 31–35

Weight	Height 5'2"	5'3"	5'4"	5'5"	5'6"	5'7"	5'8"
130	40,970	40,675	40,389	40,112	39,843	39,582	39,328
135	40,308	40,010	39,721	39,441	39,170	38,907	38,651
140	39,692	39,392	39,101	38,819	38,545	38,280	38,022
145	39,119	38,816	38,523	38,239	37,963	37,696	37,436
150	38,584	38,279	37,984	37,698	37,420	37,151	36,890
155	38,084	37,777	37,480	37,192	36,912	36,641	36,378
160	37,615	37,306	37,007	36,717	36,436	36,164	35,899
165	37,174	36,864	36,563	36,272	35,989	35,715	35,449
170	36,760	36,448	36,145	35,852	35,568	35,292	35,025
175	36,369	36,055	35,751	35,457	35,171	34,894	34,625
180	35,999	35,684	35,379	35,083	34,796	34,518	34,248
185	35,650	35,334	35,027	34,730	34,442	34,162	33,891
190	35,319	35,001	34,693	34,395	34,106	33,825	33,553
195	35,005	34,686	34,377	34,077	33,787	33,505	33,232
200	34,707	34,387	34,076	33,776	33,484	33,201	32,927
205	34,423	34,102	33,790	33,489	33,196	32,912	32,637
210	34,153	33,830	33,518	33,215	32,922	32,637	32,361
215	33,895	33,572	33,259	32,955	32,660	32,375	32,097
220	33,649	33,325	33,011	32,706	32,411	32,124	31,846
225	33,414	33,089	32,774	32,468	32,172	31,885	31,606
230	33,190	32,863	32,547	32,241	31,944	31,656	31,376
235	32,974	32,647	32,330	32,023	31,726	31,437	31,156
240	32,768	32,440	32,123	31,815	31,516	31,227	30,945
245	32,570	32,242	31,923	31,615	31,315	31,025	30,743
250	32,380	32,051	31,732	31,422	31,123	30,832	30,549
255	32,198	31,868	31,548	31,238	30,937	30,646	30,363
260	32,022	31,692	31,371	31,060	30,759	30,467	30,183
265	31,854	31,522	31,201	30,890	30,588	30,295	30,011
270	31,691	31,359	31,037	30,725	30,423	30,129	29,845
275	31,534	31,202	30,879	30,567	30,264	29,970	29,685
280	31,383	31,050	30,727	30,414	30,110	29,816	29,530
285	31,237	30,904	30,580	30,267	29,962	29,668	29,381
290	31,097	30,762	30,438	30,124	29,820	29,524	29,237
295	30,961	30,626	30,301	29,987	29,682	29,386	29,098
300	30,829	30,494	30,169	29,854	29,548	29,252	28,964
305	30,702	30,366	30,041	29,725	29,419	29,122	28,834
310	30,579	30,243	29,917	29,601	29,294	28,997	28,708

APPENDIX B

ENERGY EXPENDITURE IN BODYSTEPS
Men Ages 31–35

5'9"	5'10"	5'11"	6'0"	6'1"	6'2"	6'3"	6'4"	6'5"
39,083	38,844	38,612	38,386	38,166	37,953	37,745	37,542	37,345
38,403	38,162	37,928	37,700	37,479	37,263	37,053	36,849	36,650
37,772	37,529	37,293	37,063	36,840	36,623	36,411	36,205	36,005
37,184	36,940	36,702	36,470	36,245	36,027	35,813	35,606	35,404
36,636	36,389	36,150	35,917	35,690	35,470	35,256	35,047	34,843
36,123	35,875	35,634	35,399	35,171	34,949	34,734	34,523	34,319
35,642	35,392	35,150	34,914	34,685	34,461	34,244	34,033	33,827
35,190	34,939	34,695	34,458	34,227	34,003	33,785	33,572	33,365
34,765	34,513	34,268	34,029	33,797	33,572	33,352	33,138	32,930
34,364	34,111	33,864	33,625	33,391	33,165	32,944	32,729	32,520
33,986	33,731	33,483	33,242	33,008	32,780	32,559	32,343	32,133
33,627	33,372	33,123	32,881	32,646	32,417	32,194	31,977	31,766
33,288	33,031	32,781	32,539	32,302	32,073	31,849	31,631	31,419
32,966	32,708	32,457	32,214	31,977	31,746	31,522	31,303	31,090
32,660	32,401	32,150	31,905	31,667	31,436	31,210	30,991	30,777
32,369	32,110	31,857	31,612	31,373	31,140	30,914	30,694	30,480
32,092	31,832	31,578	31,332	31,092	30,859	30,632	30,412	30,196
31,828	31,567	31,313	31,065	30,825	30,591	30,364	30,142	29,926
31,576	31,314	31,059	30,811	30,570	30,335	30,107	29,885	29,668
31,335	31,072	30,816	30,568	30,326	30,091	29,862	29,639	29,422
31,105	30,841	30,585	30,335	30,093	29,857	29,627	29,404	29,186
30,884	30,620	30,363	30,113	29,870	29,633	29,403	29,179	28,961
30,673	30,407	30,150	29,899	29,656	29,418	29,188	28,963	28,744
30,470	30,204	29,946	29,695	29,450	29,213	28,981	28,756	28,537
30,275	30,009	29,750	29,498	29,253	29,015	28,783	28,558	28,338
30,088	29,821	29,561	29,309	29,064	28,825	28,593	28,367	28,146
29,908	29,640	29,380	29,128	28,882	28,643	28,410	28,183	27,962
29,735	29,467	29,206	28,953	28,707	28,467	28,234	28,007	27,785
29,568	29,300	29,039	28,785	28,538	28,298	28,064	27,836	27,615
29,408	29,138	28,877	28,623	28,375	28,135	27,901	27,673	27,451
29,253	28,983	28,721	28,466	28,219	27,978	27,743	27,515	27,292
29,103	28,833	28,571	28,316	28,067	27,826	27,591	27,362	27,139
28,959	28,688	28,426	28,170	27,921	27,680	27,444	27,215	26,992
28,820	28,549	28,285	28,029	27,780	27,538	27,302	27,073	26,849
28,685	28,413	28,150	27,893	27,644	27,401	27,165	26,935	26,711
28,554	28,283	28,019	27,762	27,512	27,269	27,033	26,802	26,578
28,428	28,156	27,892	27,634	27,384	27,141	26,904	26,674	26,449

ENERGY EXPENDITURE IN BODYSTEPS
Men Ages 36–40

Weight	Height 5'2"	5'3"	5'4"	5'5"	5'6"	5'7"	5'8"
130	40,323	40,041	39,768	39,503	39,245	38,996	38,754
135	39,691	39,406	39,129	38,861	38,601	38,349	38,104
140	39,104	38,816	38,536	38,265	38,003	37,748	37,501
145	38,558	38,267	37,984	37,711	37,446	37,188	36,939
150	38,048	37,754	37,469	37,193	36,926	36,666	36,414
155	37,571	37,274	36,987	36,709	36,439	36,178	35,923
160	37,123	36,825	36,535	36,255	35,983	35,720	35,464
165	36,703	36,402	36,111	35,829	35,555	35,289	35,031
170	36,308	36,005	35,712	35,427	35,152	34,884	34,625
175	35,935	35,630	35,335	35,049	34,772	34,502	34,241
180	35,583	35,276	34,979	34,692	34,413	34,142	33,879
185	35,249	34,941	34,643	34,353	34,073	33,801	33,537
190	34,934	34,624	34,324	34,033	33,751	33,478	33,212
195	34,634	34,323	34,022	33,729	33,446	33,171	32,904
200	34,350	34,037	33,734	33,441	33,156	32,880	32,612
205	34,079	33,765	33,461	33,166	32,880	32,603	32,333
210	33,822	33,506	33,201	32,905	32,617	32,339	32,068
215	33,576	33,259	32,953	32,655	32,367	32,087	31,816
220	33,341	33,024	32,716	32,417	32,128	31,847	31,575
225	33,117	32,798	32,489	32,190	31,899	31,618	31,344
230	32,903	32,583	32,273	31,972	31,681	31,398	31,124
235	32,698	32,377	32,066	31,764	31,472	31,188	30,913
240	32,501	32,179	31,867	31,564	31,271	30,987	30,710
245	32,312	31,989	31,676	31,373	31,079	30,793	30,516
250	32,131	31,807	31,493	31,189	30,894	30,608	30,330
255	31,957	31,632	31,318	31,013	30,717	30,430	30,151
260	31,790	31,464	31,149	30,843	30,546	30,259	29,979
265	31,629	31,302	30,986	30,679	30,382	30,094	29,814
270	31,474	31,147	30,829	30,522	30,224	29,935	29,654
275	31,324	30,996	30,679	30,370	30,072	29,782	29,501
280	31,180	30,852	30,533	30,224	29,925	29,634	29,352
285	31,041	30,712	30,393	30,083	29,783	29,492	29,210
290	30,907	30,577	30,257	29,947	29,646	29,355	29,072
295	30,777	30,447	30,126	29,815	29,514	29,222	28,938
300	30,652	30,321	29,999	29,688	29,386	29,093	28,809
305	30,531	30,199	29,877	29,565	29,263	28,969	28,685
310	30,414	30,081	29,758	29,446	29,143	28,849	28,564

ENERGY EXPENDITURE IN BODYSTEPS
Men Ages 36–40

5'9"	5'10"	5'11"	6'0"	6'1"	6'2"	6'3"	6'4"	6'5"
38,519	38,291	38,069	37,853	37,643	37,439	37,241	37,047	36,859
37,866	37,636	37,411	37,193	36,981	36,774	36,573	36,378	36,187
37,260	37,027	36,800	36,580	36,365	36,157	35,954	35,756	35,564
36,696	36,461	36,232	36,009	35,793	35,582	35,377	35,177	34,983
36,169	35,932	35,701	35,476	35,258	35,045	34,839	34,637	34,441
35,677	35,437	35,204	34,978	34,758	34,543	34,335	34,132	33,934
35,215	34,973	34,739	34,511	34,289	34,073	33,863	33,658	33,459
34,781	34,538	34,302	34,072	33,848	33,631	33,419	33,213	33,012
34,373	34,128	33,890	33,659	33,434	33,215	33,002	32,794	32,592
33,988	33,741	33,502	33,269	33,043	32,822	32,608	32,399	32,196
33,624	33,376	33,135	32,901	32,674	32,452	32,236	32,026	31,822
33,280	33,031	32,789	32,553	32,324	32,102	31,885	31,674	31,468
32,954	32,704	32,460	32,224	31,993	31,770	31,552	31,339	31,133
32,645	32,393	32,149	31,911	31,680	31,455	31,235	31,022	30,814
32,351	32,098	31,853	31,614	31,381	31,155	30,935	30,721	30,512
32,072	31,818	31,571	31,331	31,098	30,871	30,650	30,434	30,225
31,806	31,551	31,303	31,062	30,828	30,600	30,378	30,162	29,951
31,552	31,296	31,047	30,805	30,570	30,341	30,118	29,901	29,690
31,310	31,053	30,803	30,560	30,324	30,094	29,871	29,653	29,441
31,079	30,821	30,570	30,326	30,089	29,859	29,634	29,416	29,203
30,857	30,599	30,347	30,102	29,865	29,633	29,408	29,189	28,975
30,645	30,386	30,133	29,888	29,649	29,417	29,191	28,971	28,757
30,442	30,182	29,929	29,683	29,443	29,210	28,984	28,763	28,548
30,248	29,986	29,732	29,486	29,245	29,012	28,784	28,563	28,347
30,061	29,799	29,544	29,296	29,056	28,821	28,593	28,371	28,155
29,881	29,618	29,363	29,115	28,873	28,638	28,410	28,187	27,970
29,708	29,445	29,189	28,940	28,698	28,462	28,233	28,010	27,792
29,542	29,278	29,021	28,772	28,529	28,293	28,063	27,839	27,621
29,382	29,117	28,860	28,610	28,366	28,130	27,899	27,675	27,457
29,227	28,962	28,704	28,454	28,210	27,973	27,742	27,517	27,298
29,079	28,813	28,554	28,303	28,059	27,821	27,590	27,364	27,145
28,935	28,669	28,410	28,158	27,913	27,675	27,443	27,217	26,997
28,797	28,530	28,270	28,018	27,772	27,534	27,301	27,075	26,854
28,663	28,395	28,135	27,882	27,636	27,397	27,164	26,938	26,717
28,533	28,265	28,005	27,751	27,505	27,265	27,032	26,805	26,583
28,408	28,140	27,878	27,625	27,378	27,138	26,904	26,676	26,455
28,287	28,018	27,756	27,502	27,255	27,014	26,780	26,552	26,330

ENERGY EXPENDITURE IN BODYSTEPS
Men Ages 41–45

Weight	Height						
	5'2"	5'3"	5'4"	5'5"	5'6"	5'7"	5'8"
130	39,661	39,392	39,132	38,879	38,634	38,396	38,166
135	39,060	38,788	38,523	38,267	38,019	37,778	37,544
140	38,502	38,226	37,958	37,699	37,447	37,203	36,966
145	37,983	37,703	37,432	37,170	36,915	36,668	36,428
150	37,498	37,215	36,942	36,676	36,419	36,169	35,926
155	37,045	36,759	36,482	36,214	35,954	35,702	35,457
160	36,619	36,331	36,052	35,781	35,519	35,264	35,017
165	36,220	35,929	35,647	35,374	35,109	34,853	34,603
170	35,844	35,551	35,267	34,991	34,724	34,465	34,214
175	35,490	35,194	34,908	34,630	34,361	34,100	33,847
180	35,155	34,857	34,569	34,289	34,019	33,756	33,500
185	34,838	34,539	34,248	33,967	33,694	33,430	33,173
190	34,538	34,237	33,945	33,661	33,387	33,121	32,862
195	34,254	33,950	33,656	33,372	33,095	32,827	32,567
200	33,983	33,678	33,383	33,096	32,818	32,549	32,287
205	33,726	33,419	33,122	32,834	32,555	32,284	32,021
210	33,481	33,173	32,874	32,585	32,304	32,032	31,768
215	33,248	32,938	32,638	32,347	32,065	31,791	31,526
220	33,025	32,713	32,412	32,120	31,837	31,562	31,295
225	32,812	32,499	32,196	31,903	31,618	31,342	31,074
230	32,608	32,294	31,990	31,695	31,410	31,133	30,864
235	32,413	32,098	31,793	31,497	31,210	30,932	30,662
240	32,226	31,910	31,603	31,306	31,018	30,739	30,468
245	32,046	31,729	31,422	31,124	30,835	30,554	30,282
250	31,874	31,556	31,247	30,948	30,658	30,377	30,104
255	31,709	31,389	31,080	30,780	30,489	30,207	29,933
260	31,550	31,229	30,919	30,618	30,326	30,043	29,768
265	31,397	31,075	30,764	30,462	30,169	29,885	29,610
270	31,249	30,927	30,615	30,312	30,018	29,734	29,457
275	31,107	30,784	30,471	30,167	29,873	29,587	29,310
280	30,970	30,646	30,332	30,028	29,733	29,446	29,168
285	30,838	30,513	30,198	29,893	29,597	29,310	29,032
290	30,711	30,385	30,069	29,763	29,467	29,179	28,899
295	30,587	30,261	29,944	29,638	29,340	29,052	28,772
300	30,468	30,141	29,824	29,516	29,218	28,929	28,648
305	30,353	30,025	29,707	29,399	29,100	28,810	28,529
310	30,242	29,913	29,594	29,285	28,986	28,696	28,414

ENERGY EXPENDITURE IN BODYSTEPS
Men Ages 41–45

5'9"	5'10"	5'11"	6'0"	6'1"	6'2"	6'3"	6'4"	6'5"
37,942	37,724	37,513	37,307	37,108	36,913	36,724	36,539	36,360
37,317	37,096	36,882	36,673	36,470	36,273	36,081	35,894	35,712
36,736	36,513	36,295	36,084	35,879	35,679	35,485	35,295	35,111
36,196	35,969	35,750	35,536	35,328	35,126	34,929	34,737	34,551
35,691	35,462	35,240	35,024	34,814	34,610	34,411	34,217	34,028
35,219	34,988	34,764	34,545	34,333	34,127	33,926	33,730	33,539
34,777	34,544	34,317	34,097	33,882	33,674	33,471	33,273	33,081
34,361	34,126	33,897	33,675	33,459	33,249	33,044	32,845	32,650
33,970	33,733	33,502	33,278	33,060	32,848	32,642	32,441	32,245
33,601	33,362	33,130	32,904	32,684	32,471	32,263	32,060	31,863
33,253	33,012	32,778	32,551	32,330	32,114	31,905	31,701	31,502
32,923	32,681	32,445	32,216	31,994	31,777	31,566	31,361	31,161
32,611	32,367	32,130	31,900	31,676	31,458	31,245	31,039	30,838
32,315	32,070	31,831	31,599	31,374	31,155	30,941	30,733	30,531
32,034	31,787	31,547	31,314	31,087	30,867	30,652	30,443	30,239
31,766	31,518	31,277	31,042	30,815	30,593	30,377	30,167	29,962
31,511	31,262	31,019	30,784	30,555	30,332	30,115	29,904	29,698
31,268	31,017	30,774	30,537	30,307	30,083	29,865	29,653	29,446
31,036	30,784	30,540	30,302	30,071	29,846	29,627	29,414	29,206
30,814	30,562	30,316	30,077	29,845	29,619	29,399	29,185	28,976
30,602	30,349	30,102	29,862	29,629	29,402	29,181	28,966	28,757
30,399	30,144	29,897	29,656	29,422	29,194	28,973	28,757	28,546
30,205	29,949	29,700	29,459	29,224	28,995	28,773	28,556	28,345
30,018	29,761	29,512	29,270	29,034	28,804	28,581	28,363	28,152
29,839	29,581	29,331	29,088	28,851	28,621	28,397	28,179	27,966
29,667	29,408	29,157	28,913	28,676	28,445	28,220	28,001	27,788
29,501	29,242	28,990	28,745	28,507	28,275	28,050	27,830	27,616
29,342	29,082	28,829	28,584	28,345	28,112	27,886	27,666	27,451
29,189	28,928	28,675	28,428	28,189	27,955	27,729	27,508	27,292
29,041	28,779	28,525	28,278	28,038	27,804	27,577	27,355	27,139
28,898	28,636	28,381	28,134	27,893	27,658	27,430	27,208	26,992
28,761	28,498	28,243	27,994	27,753	27,518	27,289	27,066	26,849
28,628	28,365	28,109	27,860	27,617	27,382	27,152	26,929	26,712
28,500	28,236	27,979	27,729	27,487	27,251	27,021	26,797	26,579
28,376	28,111	27,854	27,604	27,360	27,124	26,893	26,669	26,450
28,256	27,991	27,733	27,482	27,238	27,001	26,770	26,545	26,326
28,140	27,874	27,616	27,364	27,120	26,882	26,651	26,425	26,206

THE STEP DIET

ENERGY EXPENDITURE IN BODYSTEPS
Men Ages 46–50

Weight	Height 5'2"	5'3"	5'4"	5'5"	5'6"	5'7"	5'8"
130	38,683	38,430	38,184	37,946	37,715	37,492	37,274
135	38,119	37,861	37,611	37,369	37,134	36,906	36,685
140	37,594	37,332	37,079	36,833	36,594	36,363	36,138
145	37,106	36,840	36,583	36,334	36,092	35,857	35,629
150	36,651	36,381	36,120	35,868	35,622	35,385	35,154
155	36,224	35,952	35,688	35,432	35,184	34,943	34,709
160	35,825	35,549	35,282	35,023	34,772	34,529	34,292
165	35,450	35,171	34,901	34,639	34,386	34,140	33,901
170	35,096	34,815	34,542	34,278	34,022	33,773	33,532
175	34,763	34,479	34,204	33,938	33,679	33,428	33,185
180	34,449	34,162	33,885	33,616	33,355	33,102	32,857
185	34,151	33,862	33,583	33,312	33,049	32,794	32,546
190	33,869	33,578	33,296	33,023	32,758	32,501	32,252
195	33,602	33,309	33,025	32,750	32,483	32,224	31,973
200	33,348	33,053	32,767	32,490	32,221	31,961	31,708
205	33,106	32,809	32,521	32,243	31,972	31,710	31,456
210	32,876	32,577	32,288	32,007	31,735	31,472	31,216
215	32,656	32,356	32,065	31,783	31,509	31,244	30,987
220	32,447	32,145	31,852	31,569	31,294	31,027	30,768
225	32,247	31,943	31,649	31,364	31,088	30,820	30,559
230	32,055	31,750	31,455	31,168	30,890	30,621	30,360
235	31,872	31,565	31,268	30,981	30,702	30,431	30,168
240	31,696	31,388	31,090	30,801	30,521	30,249	29,985
245	31,528	31,218	30,919	30,629	30,347	30,074	29,809
250	31,366	31,055	30,755	30,463	30,181	29,907	29,640
255	31,210	30,899	30,597	30,304	30,021	29,745	29,478
260	31,061	30,748	30,445	30,151	29,867	29,590	29,322
265	30,917	30,603	30,299	30,004	29,719	29,441	29,172
270	30,779	30,464	30,159	29,863	29,576	29,298	29,028
275	30,645	30,329	30,023	29,726	29,439	29,159	28,889
280	30,516	30,199	29,892	29,595	29,306	29,026	28,754
285	30,392	30,074	29,766	29,468	29,178	28,897	28,625
290	30,272	29,953	29,645	29,345	29,055	28,773	28,500
295	30,157	29,837	29,527	29,227	28,936	28,653	28,379
300	30,045	29,724	29,413	29,112	28,820	28,537	28,262
305	29,936	29,615	29,303	29,001	28,709	28,425	28,149
310	29,831	29,509	29,197	28,894	28,601	28,316	28,040

ENERGY EXPENDITURE IN BODYSTEPS
Men Ages 46–50

5'9"	5'10"	5'11"	6'0"	6'1"	6'2"	6'3"	6'4"	6'5"
37,063	36,858	36,659	36,465	36,277	36,094	35,915	35,742	35,572
36,471	36,262	36,059	35,862	35,671	35,484	35,303	35,126	34,954
35,920	35,708	35,502	35,302	35,108	34,918	34,734	34,554	34,380
35,408	35,193	34,984	34,781	34,584	34,391	34,204	34,022	33,845
34,930	34,712	34,500	34,294	34,094	33,900	33,710	33,526	33,346
34,482	34,262	34,047	33,839	33,637	33,440	33,248	33,061	32,879
34,063	33,840	33,623	33,412	33,208	33,008	32,814	32,625	32,441
33,669	33,443	33,224	33,012	32,805	32,603	32,407	32,216	32,030
33,298	33,070	32,849	32,634	32,425	32,222	32,024	31,831	31,643
32,948	32,719	32,495	32,279	32,067	31,862	31,662	31,468	31,278
32,618	32,386	32,161	31,943	31,730	31,523	31,321	31,125	30,934
32,306	32,072	31,845	31,625	31,410	31,201	30,998	30,800	30,608
32,010	31,775	31,546	31,324	31,107	30,897	30,692	30,493	30,299
31,729	31,492	31,262	31,038	30,820	30,608	30,402	30,201	30,006
31,462	31,224	30,992	30,767	30,547	30,334	30,127	29,924	29,727
31,209	30,969	30,735	30,508	30,288	30,073	29,864	29,661	29,463
30,967	30,726	30,491	30,263	30,041	29,825	29,615	29,410	29,211
30,737	30,494	30,258	30,028	29,805	29,588	29,376	29,171	28,970
30,517	30,273	30,035	29,804	29,580	29,362	29,149	28,942	28,741
30,307	30,061	29,823	29,591	29,365	29,146	28,932	28,724	28,521
30,106	29,859	29,619	29,386	29,159	28,939	28,724	28,515	28,312
29,913	29,665	29,424	29,190	28,963	28,741	28,525	28,315	28,111
29,729	29,480	29,238	29,003	28,774	28,551	28,335	28,124	27,918
29,552	29,302	29,059	28,823	28,593	28,369	28,152	27,940	27,734
29,382	29,131	28,887	28,650	28,419	28,195	27,976	27,764	27,557
29,219	28,967	28,722	28,484	28,252	28,027	27,808	27,594	27,386
29,062	28,809	28,563	28,324	28,092	27,866	27,646	27,431	27,223
28,911	28,657	28,410	28,171	27,937	27,710	27,490	27,274	27,065
28,766	28,511	28,263	28,023	27,789	27,561	27,339	27,123	26,913
28,626	28,370	28,122	27,880	27,645	27,417	27,195	26,978	26,767
28,490	28,234	27,985	27,743	27,507	27,278	27,055	26,838	26,626
28,360	28,103	27,853	27,610	27,374	27,144	26,920	26,702	26,490
28,234	27,976	27,726	27,482	27,245	27,015	26,790	26,572	26,359
28,113	27,854	27,603	27,358	27,121	26,889	26,664	26,445	26,232
27,995	27,736	27,484	27,239	27,000	26,769	26,543	26,323	26,109
27,881	27,621	27,369	27,123	26,884	26,652	26,425	26,205	25,991
27,771	27,511	27,257	27,011	26,772	26,539	26,312	26,091	25,876

ENERGY EXPENDITURE IN BODYSTEPS
Men Ages 51–55

Weight	Height 5'2"	5'3"	5'4"	5'5"	5'6"	5'7"	5'8"
130	37,705	37,467	37,237	37,013	36,797	36,587	36,383
135	37,177	36,934	36,699	36,471	36,249	36,035	35,827
140	36,686	36,439	36,199	35,967	35,741	35,523	35,310
145	36,229	35,978	35,734	35,497	35,268	35,046	34,830
150	35,803	35,547	35,299	35,059	34,826	34,600	34,381
155	35,404	35,145	34,893	34,649	34,413	34,184	33,961
160	35,030	34,767	34,512	34,265	34,026	33,793	33,568
165	34,679	34,413	34,155	33,904	33,662	33,427	33,198
170	34,348	34,079	33,818	33,565	33,319	33,081	32,850
175	34,037	33,764	33,500	33,245	32,997	32,756	32,522
180	33,742	33,467	33,201	32,942	32,692	32,448	32,213
185	33,464	33,186	32,917	32,656	32,403	32,158	31,920
190	33,200	32,920	32,648	32,385	32,130	31,882	31,642
195	32,950	32,667	32,393	32,128	31,871	31,621	31,379
200	32,712	32,427	32,151	31,884	31,624	31,373	31,128
205	32,486	32,199	31,921	31,651	31,390	31,136	30,890
210	32,270	31,981	31,701	31,430	31,167	30,911	30,664
215	32,065	31,774	31,492	31,219	30,954	30,697	30,448
220	31,869	31,576	31,292	31,018	30,751	30,492	30,241
225	31,682	31,387	31,102	30,825	30,557	30,297	30,044
230	31,502	31,206	30,919	30,641	30,371	30,110	29,856
235	31,331	31,033	30,744	30,465	30,194	29,930	29,675
240	31,166	30,867	30,577	30,296	30,023	29,759	29,502
245	31,009	30,708	30,416	30,134	29,860	29,594	29,336
250	30,857	30,555	30,262	29,978	29,703	29,436	29,177
255	30,712	30,408	30,114	29,829	29,552	29,284	29,024
260	30,572	30,267	29,971	29,685	29,407	29,138	28,877
265	30,437	30,131	29,834	29,547	29,268	28,997	28,735
270	30,308	30,000	29,702	29,414	29,134	28,862	28,599
275	30,183	29,874	29,575	29,285	29,004	28,732	28,467
280	30,062	29,753	29,453	29,162	28,880	28,606	28,340
285	29,946	29,635	29,334	29,042	28,759	28,485	28,218
290	29,834	29,522	29,220	28,927	28,643	28,367	28,100
295	29,726	29,413	29,109	28,816	28,531	28,254	27,986
300	29,621	29,307	29,003	28,708	28,422	28,145	27,876
305	29,519	29,205	28,900	28,604	28,317	28,039	27,769
310	29,421	29,106	28,800	28,503	28,216	27,937	27,666

APPENDIX B

ENERGY EXPENDITURE IN BODYSTEPS
Men Ages 51–55

5'9"	5'10"	5'11"	6'0"	6'1"	6'2"	6'3"	6'4"	6'5"
36,185	35,992	35,805	35,623	35,446	35,274	35,107	34,944	34,785
35,624	35,428	35,237	35,051	34,871	34,695	34,524	34,358	34,196
35,104	34,904	34,710	34,520	34,336	34,157	33,983	33,814	33,648
34,620	34,416	34,218	34,026	33,839	33,657	33,480	33,307	33,139
34,168	33,961	33,760	33,565	33,374	33,189	33,009	32,834	32,663
33,745	33,535	33,331	33,133	32,940	32,752	32,570	32,392	32,218
33,349	33,136	32,929	32,728	32,533	32,342	32,157	31,977	31,801
32,976	32,761	32,552	32,348	32,150	31,957	31,770	31,587	31,410
32,626	32,408	32,196	31,990	31,790	31,595	31,405	31,221	31,041
32,296	32,075	31,861	31,653	31,450	31,254	31,062	30,875	30,693
31,983	31,761	31,545	31,334	31,130	30,931	30,737	30,549	30,365
31,688	31,464	31,245	31,033	30,827	30,626	30,430	30,240	30,054
31,409	31,182	30,962	30,747	30,539	30,336	30,139	29,947	29,760
31,143	30,915	30,693	30,477	30,267	30,062	29,863	29,670	29,481
30,891	30,661	30,437	30,219	30,008	29,802	29,601	29,406	29,216
30,651	30,419	30,194	29,974	29,761	29,554	29,352	29,155	28,963
30,423	30,189	29,962	29,741	29,527	29,318	29,114	28,916	28,723
30,205	29,970	29,741	29,519	29,303	29,092	28,888	28,688	28,494
29,997	29,761	29,531	29,307	29,089	28,878	28,671	28,471	28,275
29,799	29,561	29,329	29,104	28,885	28,672	28,465	28,263	28,066
29,609	29,369	29,137	28,910	28,690	28,476	28,267	28,064	27,867
29,427	29,186	28,952	28,724	28,503	28,288	28,078	27,874	27,675
29,253	29,011	28,775	28,547	28,324	28,108	27,897	27,692	27,492
29,086	28,842	28,606	28,376	28,152	27,935	27,723	27,517	27,316
28,925	28,681	28,443	28,212	27,987	27,769	27,556	27,349	27,147
28,771	28,525	28,287	28,055	27,829	27,609	27,396	27,188	26,985
28,623	28,376	28,136	27,903	27,677	27,456	27,241	27,032	26,829
28,480	28,232	27,992	27,758	27,530	27,309	27,093	26,883	26,679
28,343	28,094	27,852	27,617	27,389	27,166	26,950	26,739	26,534
28,210	27,961	27,718	27,482	27,253	27,030	26,812	26,601	26,395
28,082	27,832	27,588	27,352	27,122	26,898	26,680	26,467	26,261
27,959	27,708	27,464	27,226	26,995	26,770	26,551	26,338	26,131
27,840	27,588	27,343	27,105	26,873	26,647	26,428	26,214	26,006
27,725	27,472	27,226	26,987	26,755	26,528	26,308	26,094	25,885
27,614	27,360	27,114	26,874	26,641	26,414	26,193	25,978	25,768
27,507	27,252	27,005	26,764	26,530	26,303	26,081	25,865	25,655
27,403	27,148	26,899	26,658	26,423	26,195	25,973	25,756	25,546

ENERGY EXPENDITURE IN BODYSTEPS
Men Ages 56–60

Weight	Height 5'2"	5'3"	5'4"	5'5"	5'6"	5'7"	5'8"
130	36,727	36,505	36,289	36,081	35,878	35,682	35,491
135	36,235	36,007	35,786	35,572	35,365	35,163	34,968
140	35,778	35,545	35,319	35,100	34,888	34,682	34,482
145	35,353	35,115	34,884	34,661	34,444	34,234	34,030
150	34,956	34,713	34,478	34,251	34,030	33,816	33,608
155	34,584	34,337	34,099	33,867	33,643	33,425	33,213
160	34,236	33,985	33,743	33,507	33,279	33,058	32,843
165	33,909	33,654	33,408	33,170	32,938	32,714	32,496
170	33,601	33,343	33,093	32,851	32,617	32,389	32,168
175	33,310	33,049	32,797	32,552	32,314	32,084	31,860
180	33,036	32,772	32,516	32,268	32,028	31,795	31,569
185	32,777	32,510	32,251	32,001	31,758	31,522	31,293
190	32,531	32,261	32,000	31,747	31,501	31,263	31,032
195	32,298	32,025	31,762	31,506	31,258	31,018	30,784
200	32,076	31,801	31,535	31,277	31,027	30,784	30,549
205	31,866	31,588	31,320	31,060	30,807	30,563	30,325
210	31,665	31,386	31,115	30,852	30,598	30,351	30,112
215	31,474	31,192	30,919	30,655	30,399	30,150	29,908
220	31,291	31,007	30,733	30,466	30,208	29,958	29,714
225	31,117	30,831	30,554	30,286	30,026	29,774	29,529
230	30,950	30,662	30,384	30,114	29,852	29,598	29,352
235	30,790	30,501	30,220	29,949	29,685	29,430	29,182
240	30,637	30,346	30,064	29,791	29,526	29,269	29,019
245	30,490	30,197	29,914	29,639	29,372	29,114	28,863
250	30,349	30,054	29,769	29,493	29,225	28,965	28,713
255	30,213	29,917	29,631	29,353	29,084	28,823	28,569
260	30,083	29,786	29,498	29,219	28,948	28,686	28,431
265	29,958	29,659	29,370	29,089	28,817	28,554	28,297
270	29,837	29,537	29,246	28,965	28,691	28,426	28,169
275	29,721	29,419	29,127	28,844	28,570	28,304	28,046
280	29,608	29,306	29,013	28,729	28,453	28,186	27,926
285	29,500	29,196	28,902	28,617	28,340	28,072	27,811
290	29,396	29,091	28,795	28,509	28,231	27,962	27,700
295	29,295	28,989	28,692	28,405	28,126	27,855	27,593
300	29,197	28,890	28,592	28,304	28,024	27,753	27,489
305	29,103	28,794	28,496	28,206	27,926	27,653	27,389
310	29,011	28,702	28,402	28,112	27,830	27,557	27,292

ENERGY EXPENDITURE IN BODYSTEPS
Men Ages 56–60

5'9"	5'10"	5'11"	6'0"	6'1"	6'2"	6'3"	6'4"	6'5"
35,306	35,126	34,951	34,781	34,616	34,455	34,298	34,146	33,998
34,778	34,594	34,415	34,240	34,071	33,906	33,746	33,590	33,437
34,288	34,100	33,917	33,738	33,565	33,397	33,233	33,073	32,917
33,832	33,640	33,453	33,271	33,094	32,922	32,755	32,592	32,433
33,406	33,210	33,020	32,835	32,655	32,479	32,309	32,143	31,981
33,008	32,809	32,615	32,427	32,243	32,065	31,892	31,723	31,558
32,635	32,432	32,235	32,044	31,858	31,677	31,500	31,329	31,162
32,284	32,079	31,879	31,685	31,496	31,312	31,133	30,959	30,789
31,954	31,746	31,543	31,346	31,155	30,969	30,787	30,611	30,439
31,643	31,432	31,227	31,027	30,833	30,645	30,461	30,282	30,108
31,349	31,135	30,928	30,726	30,530	30,339	30,153	29,972	29,796
31,071	30,855	30,645	30,441	30,243	30,050	29,862	29,679	29,501
30,807	30,589	30,377	30,171	29,971	29,776	29,586	29,401	29,221
30,557	30,337	30,123	29,915	29,713	29,516	29,324	29,138	28,956
30,320	30,098	29,882	29,672	29,468	29,269	29,076	28,887	28,704
30,094	29,870	29,652	29,440	29,234	29,034	28,839	28,649	28,464
29,879	29,653	29,434	29,220	29,012	28,810	28,614	28,422	28,236
29,674	29,446	29,225	29,010	28,801	28,597	28,399	28,206	28,018
29,478	29,249	29,026	28,809	28,598	28,393	28,194	27,999	27,810
29,291	29,060	28,836	28,618	28,405	28,199	27,998	27,802	27,611
29,112	28,880	28,654	28,434	28,221	28,013	27,810	27,613	27,422
28,941	28,707	28,480	28,259	28,044	27,835	27,631	27,433	27,240
28,777	28,541	28,313	28,090	27,874	27,664	27,459	27,260	27,065
28,619	28,383	28,153	27,929	27,712	27,500	27,294	27,093	26,898
28,468	28,230	27,999	27,774	27,555	27,343	27,136	26,934	26,738
28,323	28,084	27,851	27,625	27,405	27,192	26,983	26,781	26,583
28,183	27,943	27,709	27,482	27,261	27,046	26,837	26,633	26,435
28,049	27,807	27,573	27,344	27,123	26,907	26,696	26,492	26,292
27,919	27,677	27,441	27,212	26,989	26,772	26,561	26,355	26,155
27,795	27,551	27,314	27,084	26,860	26,642	26,430	26,224	26,023
27,674	27,430	27,192	26,961	26,736	26,517	26,304	26,097	25,895
27,558	27,313	27,074	26,842	26,616	26,396	26,183	25,974	25,772
27,446	27,200	26,960	26,727	26,500	26,280	26,065	25,856	25,653
27,338	27,091	26,850	26,616	26,389	26,167	25,952	25,742	25,538
27,234	26,985	26,744	26,509	26,281	26,059	25,842	25,632	25,427
27,132	26,883	26,641	26,405	26,176	25,953	25,736	25,525	25,319
27,034	26,784	26,541	26,305	26,075	25,851	25,634	25,422	25,215

ENERGY EXPENDITURE IN BODYSTEPS
Men Ages 61–65

Weight	Height 5'2"	5'3"	5'4"	5'5"	5'6"	5'7"	5'8"
130	35,749	35,543	35,342	35,148	34,959	34,777	34,599
135	35,294	35,080	34,874	34,674	34,480	34,292	34,109
140	34,870	34,651	34,440	34,234	34,035	33,842	33,654
145	34,476	34,252	34,035	33,825	33,621	33,423	33,231
150	34,108	33,879	33,657	33,442	33,234	33,032	32,835
155	33,764	33,530	33,304	33,085	32,872	32,666	32,466
160	33,441	33,203	32,973	32,750	32,533	32,323	32,119
165	33,138	32,896	32,662	32,435	32,214	32,001	31,793
170	32,853	32,607	32,369	32,138	31,914	31,697	31,487
175	32,584	32,334	32,093	31,859	31,632	31,411	31,198
180	32,330	32,077	31,832	31,595	31,365	31,141	30,925
185	32,089	31,833	31,585	31,345	31,112	30,886	30,666
190	31,862	31,603	31,352	31,109	30,873	30,644	30,422
195	31,646	31,384	31,130	30,884	30,646	30,414	30,190
200	31,441	31,176	30,920	30,671	30,430	30,196	29,969
205	31,245	30,978	30,719	30,468	30,225	29,989	29,759
210	31,060	30,790	30,528	30,275	30,029	29,791	29,560
215	30,882	30,610	30,346	30,091	29,843	29,603	29,369
220	30,713	30,439	30,173	29,915	29,665	29,423	29,187
225	30,552	30,275	30,007	29,747	29,495	29,251	29,014
230	30,397	30,118	29,848	29,587	29,333	29,087	28,848
235	30,249	29,968	29,696	29,433	29,177	28,929	28,689
240	30,107	29,824	29,551	29,285	29,028	28,778	28,536
245	29,971	29,686	29,411	29,144	28,885	28,634	28,390
250	29,840	29,554	29,277	29,008	28,748	28,495	28,249
255	29,715	29,427	29,148	28,878	28,616	28,361	28,115
260	29,594	29,305	29,024	28,752	28,489	28,233	27,985
265	29,478	29,187	28,905	28,632	28,367	28,110	27,860
270	29,366	29,073	28,790	28,515	28,249	27,991	27,740
275	29,258	28,964	28,679	28,403	28,136	27,876	27,624
280	29,154	28,859	28,573	28,295	28,027	27,766	27,512
285	29,054	28,757	28,470	28,191	27,921	27,659	27,405
290	28,957	28,659	28,371	28,091	27,819	27,556	27,301
295	28,864	28,564	28,275	27,994	27,721	27,457	27,200
300	28,773	28,473	28,182	27,900	27,626	27,361	27,103
305	28,686	28,384	28,092	27,809	27,534	27,268	27,009
310	28,601	28,298	28,005	27,721	27,445	27,178	26,918

ENERGY EXPENDITURE IN BODYSTEPS
Men Ages 61–65

5'9"	5'10"	5'11"	6'0"	6'1"	6'2"	6'3"	6'4"	6'5"
34,427	34,260	34,097	33,939	33,785	33,636	33,490	33,348	33,210
33,932	33,760	33,592	33,430	33,271	33,117	32,967	32,821	32,679
33,472	33,295	33,124	32,956	32,794	32,636	32,482	32,332	32,186
33,044	32,863	32,687	32,516	32,350	32,188	32,030	31,876	31,727
32,645	32,460	32,280	32,105	31,935	31,769	31,608	31,451	31,298
32,271	32,082	31,899	31,720	31,547	31,378	31,214	31,054	30,898
31,921	31,729	31,542	31,360	31,183	31,011	30,844	30,681	30,522
31,592	31,396	31,206	31,021	30,841	30,666	30,496	30,330	30,169
31,282	31,083	30,890	30,702	30,520	30,342	30,169	30,001	29,837
30,990	30,788	30,592	30,402	30,217	30,036	29,861	29,690	29,523
30,714	30,510	30,311	30,118	29,930	29,747	29,569	29,396	29,228
30,453	30,246	30,045	29,849	29,659	29,474	29,294	29,119	28,948
30,206	29,997	29,793	29,595	29,403	29,215	29,033	28,855	28,683
29,972	29,760	29,554	29,354	29,159	28,970	28,785	28,606	28,431
29,749	29,535	29,327	29,124	28,928	28,736	28,550	28,369	28,192
29,537	29,321	29,111	28,906	28,708	28,514	28,326	28,143	27,965
29,335	29,117	28,905	28,699	28,498	28,303	28,113	27,928	27,748
29,143	28,923	28,709	28,501	28,298	28,102	27,910	27,724	27,542
28,959	28,737	28,521	28,312	28,108	27,909	27,716	27,528	27,345
28,783	28,560	28,342	28,131	27,925	27,725	27,531	27,341	27,157
28,616	28,390	28,171	27,958	27,751	27,550	27,353	27,162	26,976
28,455	28,228	28,007	27,793	27,584	27,381	27,184	26,991	26,804
28,301	28,072	27,850	27,634	27,424	27,220	27,021	26,827	26,639
28,153	27,923	27,700	27,482	27,271	27,065	26,865	26,670	26,480
28,011	27,780	27,555	27,336	27,124	26,917	26,715	26,519	26,328
27,875	27,642	27,416	27,196	26,982	26,774	26,571	26,374	26,182
27,744	27,510	27,282	27,061	26,846	26,637	26,433	26,235	26,041
27,618	27,382	27,154	26,931	26,715	26,505	26,300	26,100	25,906
27,496	27,260	27,030	26,806	26,589	26,377	26,172	25,971	25,776
27,379	27,142	26,911	26,686	26,467	26,255	26,048	25,847	25,650
27,267	27,028	26,796	26,570	26,350	26,137	25,929	25,726	25,529
27,158	26,918	26,685	26,458	26,237	26,023	25,814	25,611	25,413
27,053	26,812	26,577	26,350	26,128	25,913	25,703	25,499	25,300
26,951	26,709	26,474	26,245	26,023	25,806	25,596	25,391	25,191
26,853	26,610	26,374	26,144	25,921	25,703	25,492	25,286	25,086
26,758	26,514	26,277	26,046	25,822	25,604	25,392	25,185	24,984
26,666	26,421	26,183	25,952	25,727	25,508	25,295	25,087	24,885

ENERGY EXPENDITURE IN BODYSTEPS
Men Ages 66–70

Weight	Height 5'2"	5'3"	5'4"	5'5"	5'6"	5'7"	5'8"
130	34,772	34,580	34,395	34,215	34,041	33,872	33,708
135	34,352	34,154	33,962	33,776	33,596	33,421	33,251
140	33,962	33,758	33,560	33,368	33,182	33,002	32,826
145	33,599	33,389	33,186	32,988	32,797	32,612	32,431
150	33,260	33,045	32,836	32,634	32,438	32,247	32,063
155	32,944	32,723	32,509	32,302	32,102	31,907	31,718
160	32,647	32,421	32,203	31,992	31,787	31,588	31,394
165	32,368	32,138	31,915	31,700	31,491	31,288	31,091
170	32,105	31,871	31,644	31,425	31,212	31,005	30,805
175	31,857	31,619	31,389	31,166	30,949	30,739	30,535
180	31,623	31,382	31,148	30,921	30,701	30,488	30,281
185	31,402	31,157	30,920	30,690	30,466	30,250	30,040
190	31,193	30,944	30,704	30,470	30,244	30,025	29,812
195	30,994	30,742	30,499	30,262	30,033	29,811	29,595
200	30,805	30,550	30,304	30,065	29,833	29,608	29,390
205	30,625	30,368	30,118	29,877	29,642	29,415	29,194
210	30,454	30,194	29,942	29,698	29,461	29,231	29,008
215	30,291	30,028	29,774	29,527	29,288	29,055	28,830
220	30,135	29,870	29,613	29,364	29,122	28,888	28,661
225	29,986	29,719	29,460	29,208	28,965	28,728	28,499
230	29,844	29,574	29,313	29,059	28,814	28,575	28,344
235	29,708	29,436	29,172	28,917	28,669	28,429	28,195
240	29,577	29,303	29,037	28,780	28,530	28,288	28,053
245	29,452	29,176	28,908	28,649	28,397	28,153	27,917
250	29,332	29,054	28,784	28,523	28,270	28,024	27,786
255	29,216	28,936	28,665	28,402	28,147	27,900	27,660
260	29,105	28,823	28,550	28,286	28,029	27,781	27,539
265	28,998	28,715	28,440	28,174	27,916	27,666	27,423
270	28,895	28,610	28,334	28,066	27,807	27,555	27,311
275	28,796	28,509	28,232	27,962	27,702	27,448	27,203
280	28,700	28,412	28,133	27,862	27,600	27,345	27,098
285	28,608	28,318	28,038	27,766	27,502	27,246	26,998
290	28,519	28,228	27,946	27,673	27,408	27,150	26,901
295	28,433	28,140	27,857	27,582	27,316	27,058	26,807
300	28,349	28,056	27,771	27,495	27,228	26,968	26,717
305	28,269	27,974	27,688	27,411	27,142	26,882	26,629
310	28,191	27,895	27,608	27,330	27,060	26,798	26,544

ENERGY EXPENDITURE IN BODYSTEPS
Men Ages 66–70

5'9"	5'10"	5'11"	6'0"	6'1"	6'2"	6'3"	6'4"	6'5"
33,548	33,394	33,243	33,097	32,955	32,816	32,682	32,550	32,423
33,086	32,926	32,770	32,619	32,471	32,328	32,189	32,053	31,921
32,656	32,491	32,331	32,175	32,023	31,875	31,731	31,591	31,455
32,257	32,087	31,922	31,761	31,605	31,453	31,305	31,161	31,021
31,883	31,709	31,540	31,375	31,215	31,059	30,908	30,760	30,616
31,534	31,356	31,183	31,014	30,850	30,691	30,536	30,384	30,237
31,207	31,025	30,848	30,676	30,508	30,345	30,187	30,032	29,882
30,899	30,714	30,533	30,358	30,187	30,021	29,859	29,702	29,548
30,610	30,421	30,237	30,058	29,885	29,715	29,551	29,391	29,234
30,337	30,145	29,958	29,776	29,600	29,428	29,260	29,097	28,938
30,080	29,884	29,694	29,510	29,330	29,156	28,986	28,820	28,659
29,836	29,638	29,445	29,258	29,076	28,898	28,726	28,558	28,394
29,605	29,404	29,209	29,019	28,834	28,655	28,480	28,310	28,144
29,386	29,182	28,985	28,792	28,605	28,423	28,246	28,074	27,906
29,178	28,972	28,772	28,577	28,388	28,204	28,025	27,850	27,680
28,980	28,771	28,569	28,372	28,181	27,995	27,814	27,637	27,465
28,791	28,581	28,376	28,177	27,984	27,796	27,613	27,434	27,261
28,611	28,399	28,192	27,992	27,796	27,606	27,421	27,241	27,066
28,440	28,225	28,017	27,814	27,617	27,425	27,238	27,057	26,880
28,276	28,059	27,849	27,644	27,446	27,252	27,064	26,880	26,702
28,119	27,901	27,689	27,482	27,282	27,086	26,897	26,712	26,531
27,969	27,749	27,535	27,327	27,125	26,928	26,737	26,550	26,368
27,825	27,603	27,388	27,178	26,974	26,776	26,583	26,395	26,212
27,687	27,463	27,246	27,035	26,830	26,630	26,436	26,247	26,062
27,554	27,329	27,111	26,898	26,692	26,491	26,295	26,104	25,919
27,427	27,201	26,981	26,767	26,559	26,356	26,159	25,967	25,781
27,305	27,077	26,855	26,640	26,431	26,227	26,029	25,836	25,648
27,187	26,958	26,735	26,518	26,308	26,103	25,903	25,709	25,520
27,073	26,843	26,619	26,401	26,189	25,983	25,782	25,587	25,397
26,964	26,732	26,507	26,288	26,075	25,868	25,666	25,469	25,278
26,859	26,626	26,399	26,179	25,965	25,756	25,554	25,356	25,164
26,757	26,523	26,295	26,074	25,858	25,649	25,445	25,247	25,053
26,659	26,423	26,194	25,972	25,756	25,545	25,341	25,141	24,947
26,564	26,327	26,097	25,874	25,657	25,445	25,239	25,039	24,844
26,472	26,234	26,004	25,779	25,561	25,348	25,142	24,940	24,744
26,383	26,145	25,913	25,687	25,468	25,255	25,047	24,845	24,648
26,297	26,058	25,825	25,599	25,378	25,164	24,956	24,753	24,555

ENERGY EXPENDITURE IN BODYSTEPS
Men Ages 71–75

Weight	Height 5'2"	5'3"	5'4"	5'5"	5'6"	5'7"	5'8"
130	33,794	33,618	33,447	33,282	33,122	32,967	32,816
135	33,410	33,227	33,050	32,878	32,711	32,549	32,392
140	33,054	32,864	32,680	32,502	32,329	32,161	31,998
145	32,722	32,526	32,336	32,152	31,973	31,800	31,632
150	32,413	32,211	32,015	31,826	31,642	31,463	31,290
155	32,123	31,916	31,715	31,520	31,331	31,148	30,970
160	31,852	31,639	31,433	31,234	31,040	30,852	30,670
165	31,597	31,380	31,169	30,965	30,767	30,575	30,388
170	31,357	31,135	30,920	30,712	30,509	30,313	30,123
175	31,131	30,905	30,685	30,473	30,267	30,067	29,873
180	30,917	30,687	30,464	30,247	30,038	29,834	29,637
185	30,715	30,481	30,254	30,034	29,821	29,614	29,413
190	30,524	30,286	30,055	29,832	29,616	29,406	29,202
195	30,342	30,101	29,867	29,640	29,421	29,208	29,001
200	30,169	29,925	29,688	29,458	29,236	29,020	28,810
205	30,005	29,758	29,518	29,285	29,060	28,841	28,629
210	29,849	29,598	29,355	29,120	28,892	28,671	28,456
215	29,700	29,446	29,201	28,963	28,732	28,508	28,291
220	29,557	29,301	29,053	28,813	28,580	28,353	28,134
225	29,421	29,163	28,912	28,669	28,434	28,205	27,983
230	29,291	29,030	28,777	28,532	28,294	28,064	27,840
235	29,167	28,903	28,648	28,401	28,161	27,928	27,702
240	29,048	28,782	28,524	28,275	28,033	27,798	27,570
245	28,933	28,665	28,406	28,154	27,910	27,673	27,444
250	28,823	28,553	28,292	28,038	27,792	27,554	27,322
255	28,718	28,446	28,182	27,927	27,679	27,439	27,205
260	28,616	28,342	28,077	27,820	27,570	27,328	27,093
265	28,518	28,243	27,975	27,716	27,465	27,222	26,985
270	28,424	28,147	27,878	27,617	27,364	27,119	26,881
275	28,334	28,054	27,784	27,522	27,267	27,021	26,781
280	28,246	27,965	27,693	27,429	27,174	26,925	26,684
285	28,162	27,879	27,606	27,340	27,083	26,833	26,591
290	28,080	27,796	27,521	27,254	26,996	26,745	26,501
295	28,002	27,716	27,440	27,171	26,911	26,659	26,414
300	27,926	27,639	27,361	27,091	26,830	26,576	26,330
305	27,852	27,564	27,284	27,014	26,751	26,496	26,249
310	27,781	27,491	27,210	26,938	26,675	26,419	26,170

ENERGY EXPENDITURE IN BODYSTEPS
Men Ages 71–75

5'9"	5'10"	5'11"	6'0"	6'1"	6'2"	6'3"	6'4"	6'5"
32,670	32,527	32,389	32,255	32,124	31,997	31,873	31,753	31,635
32,240	32,092	31,948	31,808	31,672	31,539	31,410	31,285	31,163
31,840	31,687	31,538	31,393	31,251	31,114	30,981	30,850	30,724
31,469	31,310	31,156	31,006	30,860	30,718	30,580	30,446	30,315
31,122	30,958	30,800	30,645	30,495	30,349	30,207	30,068	29,934
30,797	30,629	30,466	30,308	30,154	30,004	29,858	29,715	29,577
30,493	30,321	30,154	29,991	29,833	29,680	29,530	29,384	29,242
30,207	30,031	29,860	29,694	29,533	29,375	29,222	29,073	28,928
29,938	29,759	29,584	29,414	29,249	29,089	28,933	28,781	28,632
29,684	29,501	29,324	29,151	28,983	28,819	28,660	28,505	28,353
29,445	29,259	29,078	28,902	28,730	28,564	28,402	28,244	28,090
29,218	29,029	28,845	28,666	28,492	28,323	28,158	27,997	27,841
29,004	28,811	28,624	28,443	28,266	28,094	27,927	27,764	27,605
28,800	28,605	28,415	28,231	28,052	27,877	27,707	27,542	27,381
28,607	28,409	28,217	28,030	27,848	27,671	27,499	27,332	27,168
28,422	28,222	28,028	27,838	27,654	27,475	27,301	27,131	26,966
28,247	28,045	27,848	27,656	27,470	27,289	27,112	26,941	26,773
28,080	27,875	27,676	27,482	27,294	27,111	26,932	26,759	26,590
27,921	27,713	27,512	27,316	27,126	26,941	26,761	26,585	26,414
27,768	27,559	27,356	27,158	26,966	26,779	26,597	26,419	26,247
27,622	27,411	27,206	27,006	26,812	26,623	26,440	26,261	26,086
27,483	27,270	27,062	26,861	26,665	26,475	26,289	26,109	25,933
27,349	27,134	26,925	26,722	26,524	26,332	26,145	25,963	25,786
27,221	27,004	26,793	26,589	26,389	26,196	26,007	25,823	25,645
27,097	26,879	26,667	26,460	26,260	26,065	25,874	25,689	25,509
26,979	26,759	26,545	26,337	26,135	25,939	25,747	25,561	25,379
26,865	26,644	26,428	26,219	26,015	25,817	25,625	25,437	25,254
26,756	26,533	26,316	26,105	25,900	25,701	25,507	25,318	25,134
26,650	26,426	26,208	25,995	25,789	25,588	25,393	25,203	25,018
26,549	26,323	26,103	25,890	25,682	25,480	25,284	25,092	24,906
26,451	26,223	26,003	25,788	25,579	25,376	25,178	24,986	24,798
26,356	26,128	25,905	25,690	25,480	25,275	25,076	24,883	24,694
26,265	26,035	25,812	25,595	25,383	25,178	24,978	24,783	24,594
26,177	25,946	25,721	25,503	25,291	25,084	24,883	24,687	24,497
26,091	25,859	25,634	25,414	25,201	24,993	24,791	24,595	24,403
26,009	25,776	25,549	25,328	25,114	24,906	24,703	24,505	24,312
25,929	25,695	25,467	25,245	25,030	24,821	24,617	24,418	24,225

ENERGY EXPENDITURE IN BODYSTEPS
Men Ages 76–80

Weight	Height 5'2"	5'3"	5'4"	5'5"	5'6"	5'7"	5'8"
130	32,816	32,655	32,500	32,349	32,203	32,062	31,924
135	32,468	32,300	32,137	31,979	31,826	31,678	31,534
140	32,146	31,970	31,800	31,636	31,476	31,321	31,171
145	31,846	31,663	31,487	31,316	31,150	30,989	30,833
150	31,565	31,377	31,194	31,017	30,845	30,679	30,517
155	31,303	31,109	30,920	30,738	30,561	30,389	30,222
160	31,057	30,857	30,664	30,476	30,294	30,117	29,946
165	30,827	30,621	30,423	30,230	30,043	29,862	29,686
170	30,609	30,399	30,196	29,998	29,807	29,621	29,441
175	30,404	30,190	29,982	29,780	29,584	29,395	29,211
180	30,211	29,992	29,779	29,574	29,374	29,181	28,993
185	30,028	29,805	29,588	29,379	29,175	28,978	28,787
190	29,854	29,627	29,407	29,194	28,987	28,786	28,592
195	29,690	29,459	29,235	29,019	28,808	28,604	28,406
200	29,534	29,299	29,072	28,852	28,639	28,431	28,231
205	29,385	29,147	28,917	28,694	28,477	28,267	28,063
210	29,243	29,002	28,769	28,543	28,323	28,110	27,904
215	29,108	28,864	28,628	28,399	28,177	27,961	27,752
220	28,980	28,733	28,493	28,262	28,037	27,819	27,607
225	28,856	28,607	28,365	28,130	27,903	27,682	27,468
230	28,739	28,486	28,242	28,005	27,775	27,552	27,336
235	28,626	28,371	28,124	27,885	27,653	27,427	27,209
240	28,518	28,260	28,011	27,769	27,535	27,308	27,087
245	28,414	28,154	27,903	27,659	27,423	27,193	26,970
250	28,315	28,053	27,799	27,553	27,314	27,083	26,858
255	28,219	27,955	27,699	27,451	27,211	26,977	26,751
260	28,127	27,861	27,603	27,353	27,111	26,876	26,647
265	28,039	27,770	27,511	27,259	27,015	26,778	26,548
270	27,953	27,683	27,422	27,168	26,922	26,684	26,452
275	27,871	27,599	27,336	27,081	26,833	26,593	26,360
280	27,792	27,518	27,253	26,996	26,747	26,505	26,270
285	27,716	27,440	27,173	26,915	26,664	26,421	26,185
290	27,642	27,365	27,096	26,836	26,584	26,339	26,102
295	27,571	27,292	27,022	26,760	26,507	26,260	26,021
300	27,502	27,222	26,950	26,687	26,432	26,184	25,944
305	27,435	27,154	26,881	26,616	26,359	26,110	25,869
310	27,371	27,088	26,813	26,547	26,289	26,039	25,796

ENERGY EXPENDITURE IN BODYSTEPS
Men Ages 76–80

5'9"	5'10"	5'11"	6'0"	6'1"	6'2"	6'3"	6'4"	6'5"
31,791	31,661	31,535	31,413	31,294	31,178	31,065	30,955	30,848
31,394	31,257	31,125	30,997	30,872	30,750	30,632	30,517	30,404
31,024	30,883	30,745	30,611	30,480	30,353	30,230	30,110	29,993
30,681	30,534	30,390	30,251	30,116	29,984	29,856	29,731	29,609
30,360	30,208	30,060	29,915	29,775	29,639	29,506	29,377	29,251
30,060	29,903	29,750	29,602	29,457	29,316	29,179	29,046	28,916
29,779	29,617	29,460	29,307	29,159	29,014	28,873	28,736	28,603
29,515	29,349	29,188	29,031	28,878	28,730	28,585	28,445	28,308
29,266	29,096	28,931	28,770	28,614	28,462	28,314	28,170	28,030
29,032	28,858	28,689	28,525	28,366	28,210	28,059	27,912	27,769
28,810	28,633	28,461	28,293	28,131	27,972	27,818	27,668	27,521
28,601	28,420	28,245	28,074	27,908	27,747	27,590	27,437	27,288
28,402	28,219	28,040	27,867	27,698	27,533	27,374	27,218	27,066
28,214	28,027	27,846	27,670	27,498	27,331	27,168	27,010	26,856
28,035	27,846	27,662	27,482	27,308	27,139	26,974	26,813	26,657
27,865	27,673	27,486	27,304	27,128	26,956	26,788	26,625	26,467
27,703	27,508	27,319	27,135	26,956	26,781	26,612	26,447	26,286
27,549	27,351	27,160	26,973	26,792	26,615	26,444	26,276	26,113
27,401	27,202	27,008	26,819	26,635	26,457	26,283	26,114	25,949
27,260	27,058	26,862	26,671	26,486	26,305	26,129	25,958	25,792
27,126	26,922	26,723	26,530	26,343	26,160	25,983	25,810	25,641
26,997	26,790	26,590	26,395	26,206	26,021	25,842	25,667	25,497
26,873	26,665	26,463	26,266	26,075	25,888	25,707	25,531	25,359
26,754	26,544	26,340	26,142	25,949	25,761	25,578	25,400	25,227
26,640	26,429	26,223	26,023	25,828	25,638	25,454	25,275	25,100
26,531	26,317	26,110	25,908	25,712	25,521	25,335	25,154	24,978
26,426	26,211	26,001	25,798	25,600	25,408	25,220	25,038	24,860
26,325	26,108	25,897	25,692	25,493	25,299	25,110	24,926	24,747
26,227	26,009	25,796	25,590	25,389	25,194	25,004	24,819	24,638
26,133	25,913	25,699	25,492	25,290	25,093	24,902	24,715	24,534
26,043	25,821	25,606	25,397	25,193	24,996	24,803	24,615	24,433
25,955	25,732	25,516	25,305	25,101	24,902	24,708	24,519	24,335
25,871	25,647	25,429	25,217	25,011	24,811	24,616	24,426	24,241
25,789	25,564	25,345	25,132	24,925	24,723	24,527	24,336	24,150
25,710	25,484	25,263	25,049	24,841	24,638	24,441	24,249	24,062
25,634	25,406	25,185	24,970	24,760	24,556	24,358	24,165	23,977
25,560	25,331	25,109	24,892	24,682	24,477	24,278	24,084	23,894

ENERGY EXPENDITURE IN BODYSTEPS
Men Ages 81–85

Weight	Height 5'2"	5'3"	5'4"	5'5"	5'6"	5'7"	5'8"
130	31,718	31,575	31,437	31,302	31,172	31,046	30,924
135	31,411	31,260	31,113	30,971	30,833	30,700	30,570
140	31,127	30,967	30,813	30,664	30,518	30,378	30,241
145	30,862	30,695	30,534	30,377	30,225	30,078	29,935
150	30,614	30,441	30,273	30,110	29,952	29,799	29,650
155	30,383	30,203	30,029	29,860	29,696	29,537	29,383
160	30,166	29,980	29,800	29,625	29,456	29,292	29,132
165	29,962	29,770	29,585	29,405	29,231	29,061	28,897
170	29,770	29,573	29,382	29,198	29,018	28,845	28,676
175	29,589	29,387	29,192	29,002	28,818	28,640	28,467
180	29,418	29,212	29,012	28,818	28,629	28,447	28,270
185	29,257	29,046	28,841	28,643	28,451	28,264	28,083
190	29,103	28,888	28,680	28,478	28,282	28,091	27,907
195	28,958	28,739	28,526	28,321	28,121	27,927	27,739
200	28,820	28,597	28,381	28,171	27,968	27,771	27,580
205	28,689	28,462	28,243	28,030	27,823	27,623	27,429
210	28,564	28,334	28,111	27,895	27,685	27,482	27,284
215	28,445	28,211	27,985	27,766	27,553	27,347	27,147
220	28,331	28,094	27,865	27,643	27,427	27,218	27,015
225	28,222	27,983	27,750	27,525	27,307	27,096	26,890
230	28,118	27,876	27,641	27,413	27,192	26,978	26,770
235	28,019	27,773	27,536	27,305	27,082	26,865	26,655
240	27,923	27,675	27,435	27,202	26,977	26,758	26,545
245	27,832	27,581	27,339	27,103	26,875	26,654	26,439
250	27,744	27,491	27,246	27,009	26,778	26,555	26,338
255	27,659	27,404	27,157	26,917	26,685	26,459	26,241
260	27,578	27,321	27,071	26,830	26,595	26,368	26,147
265	27,500	27,241	26,989	26,745	26,509	26,279	26,057
270	27,425	27,163	26,910	26,664	26,426	26,194	25,970
275	27,352	27,089	26,833	26,586	26,346	26,113	25,886
280	27,283	27,017	26,760	26,510	26,268	26,034	25,806
285	27,215	26,948	26,688	26,437	26,194	25,957	25,728
290	27,150	26,881	26,620	26,367	26,122	25,884	25,653
295	27,087	26,816	26,553	26,299	26,052	25,813	25,580
300	27,026	26,754	26,489	26,233	25,985	25,744	25,510
305	26,968	26,693	26,427	26,170	25,920	25,678	25,442
310	26,911	26,635	26,367	26,108	25,857	25,613	25,377

APPENDIX B

ENERGY EXPENDITURE IN BODYSTEPS
Men Ages 81–85

5'9"	5'10"	5'11"	6'0"	6'1"	6'2"	6'3"	6'4"	6'5"
30,805	30,689	30,577	30,468	30,361	30,258	30,157	30,059	29,964
30,444	30,321	30,202	30,087	29,974	29,865	29,758	29,654	29,553
30,109	29,980	29,855	29,733	29,615	29,499	29,387	29,278	29,172
29,797	29,662	29,531	29,404	29,280	29,159	29,042	28,928	28,817
29,505	29,365	29,229	29,096	28,967	28,842	28,720	28,601	28,485
29,233	29,088	28,946	28,809	28,675	28,545	28,418	28,295	28,175
28,978	28,827	28,681	28,539	28,401	28,267	28,136	28,008	27,884
28,738	28,583	28,432	28,286	28,144	28,005	27,870	27,739	27,611
28,512	28,353	28,198	28,048	27,901	27,759	27,621	27,486	27,354
28,299	28,136	27,977	27,823	27,673	27,527	27,385	27,247	27,112
28,098	27,931	27,769	27,611	27,457	27,308	27,163	27,021	26,883
27,908	27,737	27,571	27,410	27,253	27,101	26,952	26,807	26,667
27,728	27,554	27,384	27,220	27,060	26,904	26,753	26,605	26,462
27,557	27,379	27,207	27,039	26,876	26,718	26,564	26,413	26,267
27,394	27,214	27,038	26,868	26,702	26,541	26,384	26,231	26,082
27,240	27,056	26,878	26,705	26,536	26,373	26,213	26,058	25,906
27,093	26,906	26,726	26,550	26,379	26,212	26,050	25,892	25,739
26,952	26,764	26,580	26,402	26,228	26,059	25,895	25,735	25,579
26,818	26,627	26,441	26,260	26,084	25,913	25,747	25,585	25,427
26,691	26,497	26,308	26,125	25,947	25,774	25,605	25,441	25,281
26,568	26,372	26,181	25,996	25,816	25,640	25,470	25,304	25,142
26,451	26,253	26,060	25,872	25,690	25,513	25,340	25,172	25,008
26,339	26,138	25,943	25,754	25,570	25,390	25,216	25,046	24,880
26,231	26,028	25,832	25,640	25,454	25,273	25,097	24,925	24,758
26,128	25,923	25,724	25,531	25,343	25,160	24,982	24,809	24,640
26,028	25,822	25,621	25,426	25,237	25,052	24,872	24,697	24,527
25,933	25,724	25,522	25,325	25,134	24,948	24,767	24,590	24,418
25,841	25,631	25,427	25,228	25,035	24,848	24,665	24,487	24,314
25,752	25,541	25,335	25,135	24,940	24,751	24,567	24,388	24,213
25,667	25,454	25,246	25,045	24,849	24,658	24,473	24,292	24,116
25,585	25,370	25,161	24,958	24,761	24,569	24,382	24,200	24,022
25,505	25,289	25,079	24,874	24,675	24,482	24,294	24,110	23,932
25,429	25,211	24,999	24,793	24,593	24,399	24,209	24,024	23,845
25,355	25,135	24,922	24,715	24,514	24,318	24,127	23,941	23,760
25,283	25,063	24,848	24,640	24,437	24,240	24,048	23,861	23,679
25,214	24,992	24,776	24,567	24,363	24,164	23,971	23,783	23,600
25,147	24,924	24,707	24,496	24,291	24,091	23,897	23,708	23,524

ENERGY EXPENDITURE IN BODYSTEPS
Men Ages 86–90

Weight	Height 5'2"	5'3"	5'4"	5'5"	5'6"	5'7"	5'8"
130	30,606	30,481	30,359	30,242	30,128	30,017	29,910
135	30,341	30,206	30,076	29,950	29,827	29,709	29,593
140	30,094	29,951	29,813	29,679	29,548	29,422	29,300
145	29,865	29,714	29,568	29,426	29,289	29,156	29,026
150	29,650	29,492	29,339	29,190	29,046	28,907	28,771
155	29,450	29,285	29,125	28,970	28,820	28,674	28,532
160	29,262	29,091	28,924	28,763	28,607	28,456	28,309
165	29,086	28,908	28,736	28,569	28,407	28,251	28,098
170	28,920	28,736	28,559	28,386	28,220	28,058	27,900
175	28,763	28,574	28,391	28,214	28,042	27,876	27,714
180	28,615	28,421	28,233	28,051	27,875	27,704	27,538
185	28,475	28,276	28,084	27,898	27,717	27,541	27,371
190	28,343	28,139	27,943	27,752	27,567	27,387	27,213
195	28,217	28,009	27,808	27,613	27,424	27,241	27,063
200	28,097	27,886	27,681	27,482	27,289	27,102	26,921
205	27,984	27,768	27,559	27,357	27,161	26,970	26,786
210	27,876	27,656	27,444	27,238	27,038	26,845	26,657
215	27,772	27,550	27,334	27,124	26,922	26,725	26,534
220	27,674	27,448	27,228	27,016	26,810	26,610	26,416
225	27,580	27,350	27,128	26,913	26,704	26,501	26,304
230	27,490	27,257	27,032	26,813	26,602	26,396	26,197
235	27,403	27,168	26,940	26,719	26,504	26,296	26,094
240	27,321	27,083	26,852	26,628	26,411	26,200	25,996
245	27,242	27,001	26,767	26,541	26,321	26,020	25,811
250	27,166	26,922	26,686	26,377	26,152	25,935	25,724
255	27,093	26,846	26,608	26,299	26,073	25,853	25,640
260	27,022	26,774	26,533	26,225	25,996	25,775	25,559
265	26,955	26,704	26,461	26,225	25,923	25,699	25,482
270	26,890	26,636	26,391	26,153	25,852	25,626	25,407
275	26,827	26,571	26,324	26,084	25,783	25,556	25,335
280	26,766	26,509	26,259	26,018	25,717	25,488	25,266
285	26,708	26,448	26,197	25,953	25,717	25,422	25,198
290	26,652	26,390	26,137	25,891	25,653	25,359	25,133
295	26,597	26,334	26,079	25,831	25,592	25,298	25,071
300	26,544	26,279	26,022	25,774	25,532	25,298	25,071
305	26,494	26,227	25,968	25,718	25,475	25,239	25,010
310	26,444	26,176	25,916	25,663	25,419	25,182	24,951

ENERGY EXPENDITURE IN BODYSTEPS
Men Ages 86–90

5'9"	5'10"	5'11"	6'0"	6'1"	6'2"	6'3"	6'4"	6'5"
29,805	29,704	29,606	29,510	29,417	29,326	29,238	29,152	29,069
29,482	29,373	29,267	29,164	29,065	28,967	28,873	28,781	28,691
29,181	29,065	28,953	28,844	28,738	28,634	28,534	28,436	28,340
28,901	28,779	28,660	28,545	28,433	28,324	28,218	28,115	28,014
28,639	28,512	28,387	28,266	28,149	28,034	27,923	27,815	27,709
28,395	28,261	28,132	28,006	27,883	27,764	27,647	27,534	27,424
28,166	28,027	27,892	27,761	27,634	27,510	27,389	27,271	27,157
27,950	27,807	27,667	27,532	27,400	27,271	27,146	27,024	26,906
27,748	27,600	27,455	27,315	27,179	27,047	26,918	26,792	26,670
27,557	27,404	27,256	27,112	26,971	26,835	26,702	26,573	26,447
27,376	27,220	27,067	26,919	26,775	26,635	26,499	26,366	26,236
27,206	27,045	26,889	26,737	26,589	26,446	26,306	26,170	26,037
27,044	26,880	26,720	26,565	26,414	26,267	26,124	25,984	25,849
26,890	26,723	26,560	26,401	26,247	26,097	25,951	25,808	25,670
26,745	26,574	26,407	26,246	26,088	25,935	25,786	25,641	25,500
26,606	26,432	26,262	26,098	25,938	25,782	25,630	25,482	25,338
26,474	26,297	26,124	25,957	25,794	25,635	25,481	25,331	25,184
26,348	26,168	25,993	25,823	25,657	25,496	25,339	25,186	25,038
26,228	26,045	25,867	25,694	25,526	25,363	25,204	25,049	24,898
26,113	25,928	25,747	25,572	25,401	25,236	25,074	24,917	24,764
26,003	25,815	25,633	25,455	25,282	25,114	24,950	24,791	24,636
25,898	25,708	25,523	25,343	25,168	24,997	24,832	24,670	24,513
25,797	25,605	25,417	25,235	25,058	24,886	24,718	24,555	24,395
25,701	25,506	25,316	25,132	24,953	24,779	24,609	24,444	24,283
25,608	25,411	25,219	25,033	24,852	24,676	24,504	24,337	24,175
25,519	25,320	25,126	24,938	24,755	24,577	24,404	24,235	24,071
25,433	25,232	25,037	24,847	24,662	24,482	24,307	24,137	23,971
25,351	25,148	24,950	24,759	24,572	24,391	24,214	24,042	23,874
25,271	25,066	24,867	24,674	24,486	24,303	24,124	23,951	23,782
25,195	24,988	24,787	24,592	24,402	24,218	24,038	23,863	23,693
25,121	24,913	24,710	24,513	24,322	24,136	23,955	23,778	23,606
25,050	24,840	24,636	24,437	24,245	24,057	23,874	23,697	23,523
24,981	24,769	24,564	24,364	24,170	23,981	23,797	23,618	23,443
24,914	24,701	24,494	24,293	24,098	23,907	23,722	23,542	23,366
24,850	24,636	24,427	24,225	24,028	23,836	23,649	23,468	23,291
24,788	24,572	24,362	24,159	23,960	23,767	23,579	23,397	23,218
24,728	24,511	24,300	24,094	23,895	23,701	23,512	23,328	23,148

The MegaStep Value of Foods

In the following tables, we provide the MegaStep value for many common foods. To use the tables, just find the column that includes the number of steps per calorie that you get (you recalculated this after weight loss on pages 112–13). Use this column to see the MegaStep value for each food. You can use these tables in a number of ways. You might want to occasionally calculate the MegaStep value of all the foods you eat for a few days. Make sure that the total is not greater than the MegaStep value for your energy expenditure. You can also use the tables to decide between foods. For example, you might see several versions of a favorite type of food. You can choose the one with the lower MegaStep value. You can also figure out how much extra you should walk to make up for a splurge.

THE MEGASTEP VALUE OF FOODS
BREAKFAST FOODS

SERVING SIZE: I EGG, OR AS INDICATED	STEPS/CALORIE				
	<15	16–20	21–25	26–30	>30
EGGS AND EGG DISHES					
Boiled Egg	1	1	2	2	2
Deviled Egg	2	3	3	4	5
Eggs Benedict	10	15	19	23	27
Eggs Florentine	11	16	20	25	29
Fried Egg	2	3	4	5	6
Omelet, Cheese	5	6	8	10	12
Scrambled Egg	2	2	3	3	4
PANCAKES					
Pancake, Plain, Medium	1	1	2	2	3
Pancakes, Five, with Butter and Syrup	9	13	17	20	24
WAFFLES					
Waffle, Plain, 2½ oz.	3	4	6	7	8
Waffle, Frozen	1	2	2	3	3

THE MEGASTEP VALUE OF FOODS
BEEF, POULTRY, AND FISH

SERVING SIZE: AS INDICATED	STEPS/CALORIE				
	<15	16–20	21–25	26–30	>30
BEEF, 3 ounces					
Beef Brisket, Sliced	2	2	3	3	4
Beef Chuck, Blade Roast, Braised	4	5	7	8	9
Beef Cuts	2	2	3	3	4
Beef Eye of Round, Roasted	2	3	4	4	5
Beef Flank, Braised	3	4	5	6	7
Beef, Ground	4	6	8	9	11
Beef Liver, Braised	2	2	3	4	5
Beef Patty, Cooked	2	3	4	4	5
Beef Porterhouse, Broiled	3	4	5	7	8
Beef Rib, Eye, Small End, Broiled	3	5	6	7	9
Beef Rib, Large End, Broiled	5	7	8	10	12
Beef Rib, Small End, Roasted (Prime Rib)	4	5	7	8	10
Beef Round, Bottom, Braised (Cube Steak)	2	3	4	5	6
Beef Shank Crosscuts, Simmered	3	4	5	6	7
Beef T-bone, Broiled	3	4	5	6	7
Beef Tenderloin, Broiled (Filet Mignon)	2	4	5	6	7
Beef Top Loin, Broiled (KC, NY Strip, Club)	2	3	4	5	6
Beef Top Round, Braised (London Broil)	2	3	4	5	6
Corned Beef, Cooked	3	4	5	6	7
COMMERCIAL BEEF PRODUCTS, 1 package					
Beef Brisket with Sauce, Chopped, *Cripple Creek*	2	3	3	4	5
Beef Chow Mein, *La Choy*	1	2	2	3	3
Beef Dinner Entrée with Mesquite, *Healthy Choice*	4	6	7	9	11
Beef Enchilada Entrée, *Swanson*	6	9	12	14	17
Beef Entrée, Chow Mein, *Michelina's*	3	5	6	7	8
Beef Entrée, Fiesta, *Right Course*	3	5	6	8	9
Beef Entrée, Mexicana, *Budget Gourmet*	7	10	13	16	18
Beef Entrée, Oriental, *Budget Gourmet*	3	5	6	8	9

APPENDIX C

THE MEGASTEP VALUE OF FOODS
BEEF, POULTRY, AND FISH (continued)

SERVING SIZE: AS INDICATED	STEPS/CALORIE				
	<15	16–20	21–25	26–30	>30
Beef Entrée, Stroganoff, Budget Gourmet	3	5	6	7	8
Beef Entrée, Sukiyaki, Top Shelf	4	6	8	9	11
Beef Entrée, with Gravy, Swanson	5	7	9	10	12
Beef Fajitas Entrée, Hudson	3	4	5	6	7
Beef Flavored Rice Dish, Rice-A-Roni	2	3	4	5	6
Beef Goulash, with Onion, Fried, Banquet	2	2	3	4	4
Beef Patty Entrée, Banquet	4	6	7	9	10
Beef Peppercorn Entrée, Lean Cuisine	3	5	6	7	9
Beef Pie Entrée, Stouffer's	6	8	10	13	15
Beef Pot Roast Entrée, Healthy Choice	4	6	8	9	11
Beef Pot Roast Entrée, Marie Callender's	3	5	6	7	9
Beef Ravioli Entrée, 99% Nonfat, Chef Boyardee	3	4	5	6	7
Beef Romanoff Entrée, Weight Watchers	3	4	5	6	8
Beef Sandwich, Manwich	4	6	7	9	10
Beef Sandwich, Barbecue, Tyson	3	4	5	6	7
Beef Sandwich with Cheese, Hot Pockets	5	7	9	10	12
Beef Stir-Fry Meal, Frozen, Budget Gourmet	3	5	6	7	9
CHICKEN, 3 ounces					
Chicken Breast, Fried	5	8	10	12	14
Chicken Breast, Roasted without Skin	2	3	4	5	6
Chicken Breast, Roasted with Skin	4	5	7	8	10
Chicken Leg, Fried	5	8	10	12	14
Chicken Leg, Roasted without Skin	2	3	4	5	6
Chicken Leg, Roasted with Skin	3	5	6	7	9
COMMERCIAL CHICKEN PRODUCTS, 1 package					
Chicken à la King Entrée	4	6	7	9	11
Chicken and Noodles, Frozen	5	7	9	11	13
Chicken and Vegetables Entrée	3	5	6	7	8
Chicken Breast Meal, Frozen	2	3	4	5	6

THE MEGASTEP VALUE OF FOODS
BEEF, POULTRY, AND FISH (continued)

SERVING SIZE: AS INDICATED	STEPS/CALORIE				
	<15	16–20	21–25	26–30	>30
Chicken Broccoli Alfredo Entrée	4	5	7	8	10
Chicken Chow Mein Entrée	3	5	6	7	9
Chicken Cordon Bleu	7	11	14	17	19
Chicken Divan Entrée	3	4	5	6	7
Chicken Enchilada Meal, Frozen	5	7	9	11	12
Chicken Entrée, Fried	4	6	8	9	11
Chicken Entrée, Honey Dijon	4	6	8	10	11
Chicken Entrée, Honey Mustard	5	7	9	11	13
Chicken Entrée, Mesquite	4	6	8	10	12
Chicken Entrée, Mexican	5	7	9	10	12
Chicken Entrée, Pie	7	10	13	15	18
Chicken Entrée, Primavera	3	5	6	7	8
Chicken Entrée, Sweet and Sour	7	10	12	15	17
Chicken Fettuccine, Entrée	4	5	7	8	10
Chicken Fettuccine, Italian	4	5	6	8	9
Chicken in Peanut Sauce Entrée	3	5	6	7	9
Chicken in Wine Sauce Entrée	3	4	5	6	7
Chicken Kiev Entrée	7	10	12	15	17
Chicken Pot Pie	8	11	14	17	20
Chicken Sandwich	6	8	11	13	16
Chicken Sandwich with Cheese	4	6	7	9	10
TURKEY, 3 ounces					
Turkey, Breast without Skin (10 oz)	5	7	10	12	14
Turkey, Ground, 85% Lean	2	3	4	5	6
Turkey, Leg without Skin (7³/₄ oz)	4	6	8	10	12
Turkey, Roasted, Light Meat	2	3	3	4	5
Turkey, Roasted, Dark Meat	2	3	4	4	5
Turkey, Wing	2	3	4	5	6

THE MEGASTEP VALUE OF FOODS
BEEF, POULTRY, AND FISH (continued)

SERVING SIZE: AS INDICATED	STEPS/CALORIE				
	<15	16–20	21–25	26–30	>30
FISH, 3 ounces					
Bass	1	2	2	3	3
Bluefish	2	3	4	5	6
Calamari, Breaded, Fried, 1 serving	5	6	8	10	12
Carp	2	3	3	4	5
Catfish	2	2	3	4	4
Cod	2	2	3	4	4
Crab	2	2	3	4	4
Flounder	2	2	3	3	4
Haddock	2	3	4	5	6
Herring	2	3	4	5	6
Lobster	2	3	3	4	5
Mackerel	2	3	4	5	6
Mussels	2	2	3	4	4
Orange Roughy	2	3	3	4	5
Oysters	1	1	1	2	2
Oysters, Fried	2	3	4	5	6
Salmon	2	3	4	4	5
Shrimp	1	2	2	3	3
Shrimp, Fried	3	4	5	6	7
Swordfish	2	3	3	4	5
Tuna	2	3	4	4	5
PORK, 3 ounces					
Ham	2	3	3	4	5
Ham Patty	3	4	5	6	7
Pork, Ground	3	4	6	7	8
Pork, Loin Chops	3	4	5	6	7
Pork, Loin Roast	3	4	5	6	7
Pork, Tenderloin	2	3	3	4	5

THE MEGASTEP VALUE OF FOODS
SIDE DISHES

SERVING SIZE: I PACKAGE, OR AS INDICATED	STEPS/CALORIE				
	<15	16–20	21–25	26–30	>30
BLACK BEAN ENTRÉE	**2**	**2**	**3**	**3**	**4**
Broccoli au Gratin Rice Dish, Less Salt	2	3	4	5	6
Broccoli Entrée, Pie	2	3	4	5	6
Brown Rice, Vegetable, ¹/2 cup	2	3	3	4	5
Corn, Sweet, with Butter Sauce, Frozen, Boxed, ¹/2 cup	1	2	2	3	3
Corn with Buttery Sauce, Frozen, ¹/2 cup	2	2	3	4	4
Couscous with Lentils, ¹/2 cup	3	4	5	6	7
Cream of Spinach Side Dish	2	3	4	4	5
Garlic Bread, I piece	2	3	4	5	6
Green Bean Casserole, Frozen, ¹/2 cup	1	2	2	3	3
Hash Browns, Frozen, ¹/2 cup	1	1	2	2	2
Honey Baked Beans, Nonfat, ¹/2 cup	1	2	3	3	4
Pasta Salad, Spicy Oriental, ¹/2 cup	3	4	5	6	7
Pilaf Entrée	3	4	5	6	7
Pilaf Florentine Entrée	4	5	7	8	10
Pita, one, with Lettuce	3	5	6	7	9
Poi	1	2	3	3	4
Pork and Shrimp Mini Egg Rolls	3	4	5	6	7
Potato au Gratin, ¹/2 cup	2	2	3	4	4
Potato, Cheddar Broccoli	4	6	8	9	11
Potato Entrée, Broccoli and Cheese	4	5	7	8	10
Potato Entrée, Broccoli and Ham	3	4	6	7	8
Potato Entrée, Cheddar	3	4	5	6	8
Potato Entrée, Sour Cream	3	4	5	6	8
Potato Entrée, Turkey	3	4	5	6	8
Potato Entrée, Vegetable	4	6	7	9	11
Potatoes O'Brien, ¹/2 cup	2	3	4	4	5

THE MEGASTEP VALUE OF FOODS
SIDE DISHES (continued)

SERVING SIZE: I PACKAGE, OR AS INDICATED	STEPS/CALORIE				
	<15	16–20	21–25	26–30	>30
Potatoes, Roasted, Red, Frozen, $^1/_2$ cup	1	2	3	3	4
Potatoes, Scalloped, $^1/_2$ cup	2	3	3	4	5
Potato Puffs, Prepared, $^1/_2$ cup	4	5	7	8	9
Potato Salad, $^1/_2$ cup	2	3	3	4	5
Potato Stroganoff Meal	3	5	6	8	9
Potato Wedges, Frozen, I oz	2	2	3	3	4
Red Beans and Rice Dish, $^1/_2$ cup	2	3	4	4	5
Rice and Chicken Stir-Fry Entrée	4	5	6	8	9
Rice and Vegetables Entrée, Hunan Style	3	5	6	7	8
Rice Dish, Chicken Flavored, $^1/_2$ cup	2	3	4	5	6
Rice Dish, Chicken with Broccoli, $^1/_2$ cup	2	3	4	5	5
Rice Dish, Fried, $^1/_2$ cup	3	4	5	7	8
Rice Dish, Herb and Butter, $^1/_2$ cup	2	3	4	5	6
Rice Dish, Long Grain and Wild, $^1/_2$ cup	2	3	4	5	5
Rice Dish, Sweet and Sour, $^1/_2$ cup	3	5	6	8	9
Rice Entrée, Mexican	1	2	2	3	3
Rice Medley, Frozen	4	5	6	8	9
Rice Pilaf Dish, $^1/_2$ cup	2	3	4	5	6
Salad with Shrimp, Eggs, Mayonnaise, $^1/_2$ cup	5	8	10	12	14
Sauerkraut, Canned, $^1/_2$ cup	0	1	1	1	1
Savory Couscous, $^1/_2$ cup	2	3	4	4	5
Soybean Entrée	2	4	5	6	7
Spanish Rice Dish, $^1/_2$ cup	2	2	3	3	4
Spinach Soufflé Side Dish, $^1/_2$ cup	2	3	3	4	5
Spudbakes, Sour Cream and Onion, $^1/_2$ cup	1	2	2	3	3
Stuffing, Harvest Vegetable and Herb, $^1/_2$ cup	2	3	3	4	5
Sweet Potatoes, Candied, Frozen, $^1/_2$ cup	3	4	6	7	8

THE MEGASTEP VALUE OF FOODS
SIDE DISHES (continued)

SERVING SIZE: 1/2 CUP OR 1 PACKAGE	STEPS/CALORIE				
	<15	16–20	21–25	26–30	>30
Three Bean Salad, Canned, 1/2 cup	1	2	2	3	3
Tomato with Angel Hair Pasta, Spicy	3	4	6	7	8
Welsh Rarebit, 1/2 cup	2	2	3	3	4
Wild Mushroom and Herb Pilaf	3	4	5	6	7

THE MEGASTEP VALUE OF FOODS
ETHNIC FOODS

SERVING SIZE: AS INDICATED	STEPS/CALORIE				
	<15	16–20	21–25	26–30	>30
CHINESE AND ASIAN DISHES					
Beef in Black Bean Sauce, 16 oz	7	10	12	15	17
Beef Satay, 17 oz	10	14	17	21	25
Beef with Broccoli, 16 oz	8	12	15	18	21
Chicken and Almonds, 18 oz	9	12	16	19	23
Chicken, Lemon, 10 oz	7	10	13	16	19
Chicken, Moo Shu, 2 wrapped crêpes	5	8	10	12	14
Chop Suey, Chicken, 20 oz	7	10	13	16	18
Chop Suey, Pork, 20 oz	9	12	16	19	22
Chow Mein, Beef or Chicken, 24 oz	12	17	22	26	31
Egg Drop Soup with Noodles, 1 cup	2	2	3	3	4
Fortune Cookie, 1 cookie	0	0	1	1	1
Lo Mein, 16 oz	8	11	14	17	20
Sweet and Sour Pork, 18 oz	12	17	22	27	31
Vegetable Combination, 6 oz	3	5	6	7	8

THE MEGASTEP VALUE OF FOODS
ETHNIC FOODS (continued)

SERVING SIZE: AS INDICATED	STEPS/CALORIE				
	<15	16–20	21–25	26–30	>30
CAJUN AND CREOLE					
Alligator, 4 oz	2	3	4	4	5
Bouillabaisse, 2 cups	5	7	9	11	13
Cajun Fried Turkey, 8 oz	8	11	14	18	21
Crawfish Bisque, 2 cups	6	9	12	14	17
Crawfish, Cooked, 2 oz	1	1	1	1	1
Creole Jambalaya, 2 cups	7	10	13	15	18
Creole Shrimp, 2 cups	6	8	10	13	15
Jambalaya, Shrimp and Crabmeat, 2 cups	7	9	12	15	17
Red Beans and Rice, 2 cups	5	7	9	11	13
FRENCH					
Brioche, 1 cake	4	5	6	8	9
Bouillabaisse, 2 cups	5	7	9	11	13
Coq au Vin, 9 oz	10	14	18	22	26
Coquilles St. Jacques, fried, 6 large	4	5	7	8	10
Crème Brûlée, 1 cup	6	8	11	13	15
Crème Caramel, 1 cup	3	5	6	7	9
Crêpes Suzette, 1 crêpe	3	4	5	6	7
Duck à l'Orange, 9 oz	10	14	18	22	26
Escargots in Garlic Butter, 6	3	4	5	6	7
Lamb Noisettes, Fried, 2 chops	6	9	12	14	17
Mousse au Chocolat, 1 cup	5	7	9	11	13
Salade Niçoise, 2 cups	6	8	10	13	15
Veal Cordon Bleu, 9 oz	8	12	15	18	21
GERMAN					
Beef Goulash, 2 cups	7	9	12	15	17
Black Forest Cake, 1 slice	5	7	9	11	13
Bratwurst, 6 oz	6	8	10	13	15
Herring, Pickled with Sour Cream, 4 oz	4	6	7	9	10

THE MEGASTEP VALUE OF FOODS
ETHNIC FOODS (continued)

SERVING SIZE: AS INDICATED	STEPS/CALORIE				
	<15	16–20	21–25	26–30	>30
Kugelhupf Cake, 1 large slice	5	7	9	11	13
Sauerbraten Pork, 1 piece	8	12	15	18	21
Wiener Schnitzel, 1 medium	9	14	17	21	25
GREEK					
Baklava Pastry, 3³/₄ oz	5	7	9	11	13
Calamari, 1 cup	4	5	7	8	10
Galactobureko, 1 piece	5	6	8	10	12
Kataifi, 8 oz	4	6	8	10	12
Moussaka, 8 oz	4	6	8	10	12
Tyropita, 1 piece	4	6	8	10	12
HAWAIIAN					
Ahi Tuna, Grilled, 6 oz	3	4	5	6	7
Chicken Katsu with Rice, 9 oz	14	20	26	31	37
Haupia, 1 piece	2	2	3	3	4
Hawaiian Sweet Bread, 1 slice	2	3	4	5	6
INDIAN AND PAKISTANI					
Alu Gosht Kari, 4 oz	8	11	14	17	20
Alu Samosa, 4 oz	2	3	3	4	5
Chicken Korma, 4 oz	6	9	12	14	17
Chicken Pilaf, 4 oz	9	13	16	20	23
Chicken Tikka, 4 oz	3	5	6	7	9
Chicken Vindaloo, 4 oz	5	7	9	11	13
Dal, 1 cup	3	4	5	6	8
Gosht Kari, 4 oz	6	8	11	13	15
Lamb Pilaf, 4 oz	7	9	12	15	17
Rogan Josh, 4 oz	6	9	12	14	17
Shahi Korma, 4 oz	5	8	10	12	14
Tandoori Chicken, Breast	3	5	6	7	9

THE MEGASTEP VALUE OF FOODS
ETHNIC FOODS (continued)

SERVING SIZE: AS INDICATED	STEPS/CALORIE				
	<15	16–20	21–25	26–30	>30
JAPANESE					
Katsu-don Pork with Rice, 10 oz	14	20	25	31	36
Miso Soup, 1 cup	1	2	2	2	3
Sukiyaki, 8 oz	5	7	9	11	13
Sushi, 1 medium piece	1	1	1	1	1
Sushi Plate, 6 pieces + rolls	5	8	10	12	14
Tempura, 3 large shrimp and veggies	4	6	7	9	11
Teppan Yaki, 10 oz	6	8	11	13	16
Teriyaki Beef, 4 oz	4	6	8	10	12
Teriyaki Chicken, 4 oz	3	5	6	7	9
Sake Wine, 3 fl. oz	1	2	3	3	4
KOSHER/DELI					
Beiglach, 1 piece	4	6	8	10	12
Blintzes, 1 piece	2	2	3	3	4
Borscht, 1 cup	1	2	2	2	3
Challah, 1 slice	1	2	2	2	3
Chopped Liver, 3 oz	1	2	3	3	4
Gefilte Fish, 1 medium piece	1	1	1	2	2
Knish, 1 piece	2	2	3	4	4
Kugel, 1 cup	2	3	3	4	5
Matzo Ball Soup, 1 cup	2	3	4	5	6
THAI					
Curry, Chicken, 1 cup	4	6	8	10	11
Pad Thai, 18 oz	12	18	23	28	33
Satay Chicken and Peanut Sauce, 1 stick	5	7	9	11	13
Spring Roll, 1 roll	1	2	3	3	4
Stir-Fried Noodles, 1 cup	3	5	6	8	9

THE MEGASTEP VALUE OF FOODS
CAKES, BROWNIES, PUDDING, PIES

SERVING SIZE: I SLICE OR PIECE	Steps/Calorie				
	<15	16–20	21–25	26–30	>30
Banana Bread	2	3	4	4	5
Brownie	2	3	3	4	5
Cake, Banana Crunch	3	5	6	7	9
Cake, Boston Cream	4	6	7	9	10
Cake, Carrot	2	3	3	4	5
Cake, Chocolate, Frosted	4	5	7	8	10
Cake, Chocolate Chip	2	3	3	4	5
Cake, Fruitcake	2	3	3	4	5
Cake, German Chocolate, Frosted	4	5	7	8	10
Cake, Lemon, Frosted	5	7	8	10	12
Cake, Pineapple Upside-Down	2	2	3	4	4
Cake, Pound	4	5	7	8	10
Cake, Vanilla Layer	2	3	3	4	5
Cake, Yellow, Frosted	3	4	5	6	8
Cheesecake	3	4	5	6	7
Cinnamon Sweet Roll	3	5	6	7	9
Coffeecake, Cinnamon	5	6	8	10	12
Donut, Cream, Yeast-Leavened	3	5	6	7	9
Donut, Glazed, Yeast-Leavened	5	7	9	10	12
Pastry, Danish, Cheese	2	4	5	6	6
Pastry, Danish, Fruit	5	7	9	10	12
Pastry, Danish, Lemon	5	8	10	12	14
Pastry, Danish, Nut	3	4	5	6	7
Pie, Apple	3	5	6	7	9
Pie, Cherry	4	5	7	8	10
Pie, Chocolate Cream	5	7	9	11	13
Pie, Coconut Cream	6	9	12	14	17
Pie, Key Lime	4	5	7	8	10
Pie, Lemon	7	9	12	15	17

THE MEGASTEP VALUE OF FOODS
CAKES, BROWNIES, PUDDING, PIES (continued)

SERVING SIZE: I SLICE OR PIECE OR ½ CUP PUDDING	STEPS/CALORIE				
	<15	16–20	21–25	26–30	>30
Pie, Mince	3	5	6	8	9
Pie, Pecan	6	8	11	13	16
Pie, Pumpkin	4	5	6	8	9
Pie, Strawberry	2	3	4	4	5
Pie, Strawberry-Rhubarb	2	3	3	4	5
Pudding, Banana, Instant, Prepared	2	3	4	4	5
Pudding, Chocolate, Prepared	2	3	4	4	5
Pudding, Coconut Cream, Prepared	2	3	4	5	6
Pudding, Lemon, Prepared	2	3	3	4	5
Pudding, Rice, Prepared	2	3	3	4	5
Pudding, Tapioca, Prepared	3	5	6	7	9
Pudding, Vanilla, Prepared	3	4	6	7	8
Puff Pastry, Frozen	2	3	4	5	6
Snack Cake, Chocodiles, I package	3	4	5	6	8
Snack Cake, Snowballs, I package	2	3	3	4	5
Snack Cake, Suzy Q's, I package	2	3	4	5	6
Snack Cake, Twinkies, I package	2	3	4	5	6

THE MEGASTEP VALUE OF FOODS
COOKIES

SERVING SIZE: 1 COOKIE	STEPS/CALORIE				
	<15	16–20	21–25	26–30	>30
Apricot-Filled Cookie	1	2	2	3	3
Butter Cookie	2	3	3	4	5
Cashew Nougat Cookie	2	3	4	5	6
Chips Deluxe Cookie, Coconut	1	1	2	2	3
Chocolate Chip Cookie	2	2	3	4	4
Chocolate Chunk Cookie	2	3	3	4	5
Chocolate Sandwich Cookie	1	1	2	2	3
Chocolate Wafer Cookie	0	0	1	1	1
Coconut Macaroon Cookie	1	2	2	3	3
Deluxe Graham Cookie	2	3	3	4	5
Fig Bar Cookie	1	1	1	2	2
Fudge Vanilla Sandwich Cookie	2	2	3	3	4
Gingersnap Cookie	2	2	3	3	4
Ladyfinger Cookie	1	1	1	1	1
Lemon Cream Cookie	2	2	3	4	4
Macadamia White Chunk Cookie	2	3	4	4	5
Milk Chocolate Chip Pecan Cookie	3	4	5	6	7
Molasses Cookie, Iced	1	2	3	3	4
Nutter Butter Cookie	2	2	3	4	4
Oatmeal Cookie	1	2	3	3	4
Old-fashioned Sugar Cookie	2	3	3	4	5
Peanut Butter Cookie	2	3	3	4	5
Pecan Shortbread Cookie	1	1	2	2	3
Raisin Cookie	1	1	2	2	3
Shortbread Cookie	2	2	3	3	4
Sugar Cookie	2	2	3	4	4

THE MEGASTEP VALUE OF FOODS
ICE CREAM AND FROZEN DESSERTS

SERVING SIZE: ¹/₂ CUP OR I PIECE	STEPS/CALORIE				
	<15	16–20	21–25	26–30	>30
Banana Split, *Dairy Queen/Brazier*	6	9	12	14	17
Cone, Twist, *Hardee's*	2	3	4	5	6
Dessert, Frozen, Arctic D'Lites, *Weight Watchers*	2	2	3	4	4
Dessert, Frozen, Chocolate Fudge, *Tofutti*	2	2	3	3	4
Dessert, Frozen, Wildberry Supreme, *Tofutti*	1	1	1	1	2
Fruit Juice Bar, All Flavors, *Welch's*	1	1	1	1	1
Ice Cream Bar, Dark Chocolate Chocolate, *Cascadian Farm*	3	4	5	6	8
Ice Cream Bar, Vanilla, *Eskimo Pie*	2	3	4	5	5
Ice Cream Cone, Vanilla, Lower Fat, *McDonald's*	2	3	3	4	5
Ice Cream Cone, Vanilla, Small, *Dairy Queen/Brazier*	2	3	3	4	5
Ice Cream, Apple Crumble, *Ben & Jerry's*	4	5	6	8	9
Ice Cream, Berries 'n Banana, Sugarless, *Baskin-Robbins*	1	1	2	2	3
Ice Cream, Black Raspberry Avalanche, *Dreyer's*	3	5	6	8	9
Ice Cream, Butter Pecan, *Ben & Jerry's*	4	5	7	8	10
Ice Cream, Butter Pecan, *Breyers*	2	3	4	5	6
Ice Cream, Call Me Nuts, Sugarless, *Baskin-Robbins*	1	2	3	3	4
Ice Cream, Cappuccino Chocolate Chunk, *Healthy Choice*	2	2	3	3	4
Ice Cream, Caramel, *Swensen's*	2	2	3	3	4
Ice Cream, Caramel Apple Crisp, Lowfat, *Swensen's*	2	2	3	4	4
Ice Cream, Caramel Bar Surprise, Nonfat, *Baskin-Robbins*	1	2	3	3	4
Ice Cream, Caramel Praline, Nonfat, *Baskin-Robbins*	2	2	3	3	4
Ice Cream, Caramel Turtle Fudge, Lowfat, *Swensen's*	2	3	3	4	5
Ice Cream, Cherries Jubilee, *Baskin-Robbins*	3	4	6	7	8
Ice Cream, Cherry Chocolate Chunk, *Healthy Choice*	1	2	3	3	4
Ice Cream, Cherry Cordial, Sugarless, *Baskin-Robbins*	1	2	2	3	3
Ice Cream, Cherry Garcia, *Ben & Jerry's*	3	5	6	7	9

THE MEGASTEP VALUE OF FOODS
ICE CREAM AND FROZEN DESSERTS (continued)

SERVING SIZE: ½ CUP OR 1 PIECE	STEPS/CALORIE				
	<15	16–20	21–25	26–30	>30
Ice Cream, Chocolate Fudge Brownie, Lowfat, Swensen's	2	2	3	3	4
Ice Cream, Chocolate Vanilla Twist, Nonfat, Baskin-Robbins	1	2	2	3	3
Ice Cream, Chocolate, Dairy Queen/Brazier	3	5	6	8	9
Ice Cream, Chocolate Chip, Baskin-Robbins	3	5	6	8	9
Ice Cream, Chocolate Chip Cookie Dough, Ben & Jerry's	3	5	6	8	9
Ice Cream, Chocolate Chip, Sugarless, Baskin-Robbins	1	2	2	3	3
Ice Cream, Chocolate Chocolate Chip, Lowfat, Swensen's	2	2	3	4	4
Ice Cream, Chocolate Fudge, Ben & Jerry's	4	5	6	8	9
Ice Cream, Chocolate Fudge, Baskin-Robbins	4	5	7	8	10
Ice Cream, Chocolate Marshmallow, Nonfat, Baskin-Robbins	1	2	3	3	4
Ice Cream, Chocolate Peanut Butter Chunks, Dreyer's	4	6	7	9	10
Ice Cream, Chocolate Wonder, Nonfat, Baskin-Robbins	1	2	2	3	3
Ice Cream, Chunky Banana, Sugarless, Baskin-Robbins	1	2	2	3	3
Ice Cream, Coconut Fudge, Sugarless, Baskin-Robbins	1	2	3	3	4
Ice Cream, Completely Nuts, Blue Bunny	2	3	4	5	6
Ice Cream, Cookies & Cream, Lowfat, Swensen's	2	2	3	4	4
Ice Cream, Cookies and Cream, Breyers	2	3	4	5	6
Ice Cream, Cookies 'n Cream, Swensen's	2	2	3	4	4
Ice Cream, Double Chocolate Chunk, Dreyer's	2	3	4	5	6
Ice Cream, Double Raspberry, Light, Baskin-Robbins	1	2	2	3	3
Ice Cream, Espresso, Light, Baskin-Robbins	1	2	3	3	4

THE MEGASTEP VALUE OF FOODS
ICE CREAM AND FROZEN DESSERTS (continued)

		STEPS/CALORIE			
SERVING SIZE: 1/2 CUP OR 1 PIECE	**<15**	**16–20**	**21–25**	**26–30**	**>30**
Ice Cream, Extra Creamy Chocolate, *Breyers*	2	3	4	4	5
Ice Cream, Extra Creamy Vanilla, *Breyers*	2	3	3	4	5
Ice Cream, French Vanilla, *Baskin-Robbins*	4	5	6	8	9
Ice Cream, Hand-Dipped, *TCBY Treats*	2	3	3	4	5
Ice Cream, Jamoca Almond Fudge, *Baskin-Robbins*	4	5	6	8	9
Ice Cream, Jamoca Swirl, Nonfat, *Baskin-Robbins*	1	2	3	3	4
Ice Cream, Jamoca, No Sugar, *Baskin-Robbins*	1	2	2	3	3
Ice Cream, Kookaberry Kiwi, Nonfat, *Baskin-Robbins*	1	2	2	3	3
Ice Cream, Lowfat, *Swensen's*	2	2	3	4	4
Ice Cream, Mint Chocolate Chip, *Breyers*	2	3	4	5	6
Ice Cream, Mint Chocolate Chip, *Dreyer's*	2	2	3	3	4
Ice Cream, Mint Chocolate Cookie, *Ben & Jerry's*	3	5	6	8	9
Ice Cream, Natural Strawberry, *Breyers*	2	2	3	4	4
Ice Cream, Peach, Nonfat, *Baskin-Robbins*	1	2	2	3	3
Ice Cream, Peanut Butter & Fudge, *Breyers*	2	3	4	5	6
Ice Cream, Peanut Butter Cream, Nonfat, *Baskin-Robbins*	1	2	2	3	3
Ice Cream, Peanut Butter Cup, *Healthy Choice*	1	2	3	3	4
Ice Cream, Phish Food, *Ben & Jerry's*	4	5	6	8	9
Ice Cream, Pineapple Cheesecake, Nonfat, *Baskin-Robbins*	1	2	3	3	4
Ice Cream, Pineapple Coconut, Sugarless, *Baskin-Robbins*	1	2	2	3	3
Ice Cream, Pink Bubblegum, *Baskin-Robbins*	3	5	6	8	9
Ice Cream, Pistachio Creme Chip, Light, *Baskin-Robbins*	2	2	3	3	4
Ice Cream, Pistachio Pistachio, *Ben & Jerry's*	3	5	6	7	8
Ice Cream, Praline, *Baskin-Robbins*	4	5	6	8	9
Ice Cream, Praline, Light, *Baskin-Robbins*	2	2	3	3	4

THE MEGASTEP VALUE OF FOODS
ICE CREAM AND FROZEN DESSERTS (continued)

SERVING SIZE: 1/2 CUP OR 1 PIECE	STEPS/CALORIE				
	<15	16–20	21–25	26–30	>30
Ice Cream, Praline Pecan, Blue Bunny	2	3	4	5	6
Ice Cream, Pralines 'n Cream, Baskin-Robbins	4	5	6	8	9
Ice Cream, Raspberry, Baskin-Robbins	2	2	3	3	4
Ice Cream, Raspberry, No Sugar, Baskin-Robbins	1	2	2	3	3
Ice Cream, Rocky Path, Light, Baskin-Robbins	2	2	3	4	4
Ice Cream, Rocky Road, Light, Weight Watchers	2	3	3	4	5
Ice Cream, Soft Serve Vanilla, Nonfat, Baskin-Robbins	2	2	3	3	4
Ice Cream, Thin Mint, Sugarless, Baskin-Robbins	1	2	2	3	3
Ice Cream, Tin Roof Sundae, Healthy Choice	2	2	3	3	4
Ice Cream, Triple Chocolate, Light, Weight Watchers	2	3	3	4	5
Ice Cream, Turtle Fudge Cake, Healthy Choice	1	2	3	3	4
Ice Cream, Vanilla, Baskin-Robbins	3	5	6	7	8
Ice Cream, Vanilla, Dairy Queen/Brazier	3	4	5	6	7
Ice Cream, Vanilla Bean, Dreyer's	2	3	3	4	5
Ice Cream, Vanilla Bean, Nonfat, Baskin-Robbins	1	2	2	3	3
Ice Cream, Vanilla Heath Bar Crunch, Ben & Jerry's	4	5	7	8	10
Ice Cream, Vanilla, Light, Swensen's	1	2	3	3	4
Ice Cream, Vanilla, Premium brand	3	4	6	7	8
Ice Cream, Vanilla, Sugarless, Baskin-Robbins	1	2	3	3	4
Ice Cream, Very Berry Strawberry, Baskin-Robbins	3	4	5	6	7
Ice Cream, Wild Berry Swirl, Breyers	2	3	3	4	5
Ice Cream, World's Best Chocolate, Ben & Jerry's	4	5	6	8	9
Ice Cream, World's Best Vanilla, Ben & Jerry's	3	5	6	7	8
Ice Dessert, Italian	1	1	1	1	2
Ice Dessert, Pineapple-Coconut	1	2	3	3	4

THE MEGASTEP VALUE OF FOODS
ICE CREAM AND FROZEN DESSERTS (continued)

SERVING SIZE: ½ CUP OR 1 PIECE	STEPS/CALORIE				
	<15	16–20	21–25	26–30	>30
Ice Milk, Vanilla Soft-Serve, Lowfat	1	2	3	3	4
Ice Pop, Frozen	1	1	1	1	2
Nondairy Dessert, Mint Carob, Rice Dream	2	2	3	4	4
Praline Caramel Dessert, Lowfat, Healthy Choice	2	3	4	5	6
Praline Toffee Crunch Parfait, Weight Watchers	2	3	4	5	6
Sherbet, Orange, Baskin-Robbins	2	2	3	3	4
Sherbet, Rainbow, Baskin-Robbins	2	2	3	3	4
Sorbet and Cream, Peach/Vanilla, Cascadian Farm	2	2	3	3	4
Sorbet & Cream, Raspberry/Vanilla, Cascadian Farm	1	2	3	3	4
Sorbet, Fruit Whip, Nonfat, Baskin-Robbins	1	1	2	2	3
Sorbet, Raspberry, Cascadian Farm	1	1	2	2	3
Sorbet, Raspberry Cranberry, Baskin-Robbins	1	2	3	3	4
Sorbet, Red Raspberry, Baskin-Robbins	2	2	3	3	4
Sorbet, Strawberry, Nonfat, Baskin-Robbins	1	2	2	3	3
Strawberry Shortcake, Dairy Queen/Brazier	7	10	12	15	18
Strawberry Sundae, Dairy Queen/Brazier	4	6	8	10	12
Sundae, Chocolate, Dairy Queen/Brazier	6	8	10	12	15
Sundae, Hot Fudge, McDonald's	4	6	8	10	11
Yogurt, Frozen, Black Cherry, Nonfat, Baskin-Robbins	1	2	3	3	4
Yogurt, Frozen, Black Forest, Swensen's	1	2	2	3	3
Yogurt, Frozen, Black Forest, Lowfat, Swensen's	1	2	3	3	4
Yogurt, Frozen, Blueberry, Swensen's	1	2	3	3	4
Yogurt, Frozen, Blueberry, Lowfat, Baskin-Robbins	2	2	3	3	4
Yogurt, Frozen, Butter Pecan, Lowfat, Swensen's	2	2	3	3	4
Yogurt, Frozen, Cheesecake, Lowfat, Baskin-Robbins	2	2	3	3	4

THE MEGASTEP VALUE OF FOODS

ICE CREAM AND FROZEN DESSERTS (continued)

SERVING SIZE: 1/2 CUP OR 1 PIECE	<15	STEPS/CALORIE 16–20	21–25	26–30	>30
Yogurt, Frozen, Cherry, Nonfat, Swensen's	1	2	2	3	3
Yogurt, Frozen, Cherry Garcia, Ben & Jerry's	2	3	4	5	6
Yogurt, Frozen, Chocolate, Swensen's	2	2	3	4	4
Yogurt, Frozen, Chocolate, Lowfat, Baskin-Robbins	3	4	6	7	8
Yogurt, Frozen, Chocolate, Nonfat, Swensen's	1	2	2	3	3
Yogurt, Frozen, Chocolate Fudge Brownie, Ben & Jerry's	2	3	4	5	6
Yogurt, Frozen, Chocolate Mint, Nonfat, Baskin-Robbins	1	2	2	3	3
Yogurt, Frozen, Coconut, Swensen's	2	2	3	3	4
Yogurt, Frozen, Coconut, Nonfat, Baskin-Robbins	2	3	4	5	6
Yogurt, Frozen, Cone, Dairy Queen/Brazier	3	5	6	7	9
Yogurt, Frozen, Dutch Chocolate, Nonfat, Baskin-Robbins	1	2	2	3	3
Yogurt, Frozen, For Heaven's Cake, Lowfat, Baskin-Robbins	2	2	3	3	4
Yogurt, Frozen, Half Baked, Ben & Jerry's	3	4	5	6	7
Yogurt, Frozen, Kahlua, Nonfat, Baskin-Robbins	1	2	2	3	3
Yogurt, Frozen, Key Lime, Nonfat, Baskin-Robbins	1	2	2	3	3
Yogurt, Frozen, Kiddie, TCBY	1	2	2	3	3
Yogurt, Frozen, Kiddie, Nonfat, TCBY	1	2	2	2	3
Yogurt, Frozen, Large, TCBY	4	6	8	10	11
Yogurt, Frozen, Large, Nonfat, TCBY	4	5	7	8	10
Yogurt, Frozen, Mango in Paradise, Nonfat, Baskin-Robbins	2	2	3	4	4
Yogurt, Frozen, Maple Walnut, Nonfat, Baskin-Robbins	1	2	2	3	3
Yogurt, Frozen, Maui Brownie Madness, Baskin-Robbins	3	5	6	7	8
Yogurt, Frozen, Mocha Chip, Lowfat, Swensen's	1	2	3	3	4
Yogurt, Frozen, Ooey Gooey Cake, Ben & Jerry's	2	3	4	5	6
Yogurt, Frozen, Peach, Nonfat, Baskin-Robbins	1	2	2	3	3

THE MEGASTEP VALUE OF FOODS
ICE CREAM AND FROZEN DESSERTS (continued)

SERVING SIZE: ½ CUP OR 1 PIECE	STEPS/CALORIE				
	<15	16–20	21–25	26–30	>30
Yogurt, Frozen, Peppermint Twist, Nonfat, Baskin-Robbins	1	2	2	3	3
Yogurt, Frozen, Phish Food, Ben & Jerry's	3	4	5	6	8
Yogurt, Frozen, Piña Colada, Nonfat, Baskin-Robbins	1	2	3	3	4
Yogurt, Frozen, Raspberry, Nonfat, Baskin-Robbins	1	2	2	3	3
Yogurt, Frozen, Strawberry, TCBY	3	4	5	6	7
Yogurt, Frozen, Strawberry, Nonfat, Baskin-Robbins	1	2	2	3	3
Yogurt, Frozen, Strawberry Sundae, Dairy Queen/Brazier	3	4	5	6	7
Yogurt, Frozen, Sugarless, Nonfat, Regular, TCBY	2	3	4	5	5
Yogurt, Frozen, Triple Chocolate, Lowfat, Swensen's	2	2	3	3	4
Yogurt, Frozen, Truly Free Café Mocha, Baskin-Robbins	2	3	3	4	5
Yogurt, Frozen, Vanilla, Swensen's	2	3	3	4	5
Yogurt, Frozen, Vanilla, Lowfat, Baskin-Robbins	2	2	3	3	4

THE MEGASTEP VALUE OF FOODS
CANDY

SERVING SIZE: 1 PIECE, 1 OUNCE OR 1 BAR	STEPS/CALORIE				
	<15	16–20	21–25	26–30	>30
Candy Bar, 100 Grand, 1.5 oz	6	8	11	13	15
Candy Bar, 3 Musketeers, 1.8 oz	3	4	6	7	8
Candy Bar, Baby Ruth, 2.1 oz	4	5	7	8	10
Candy Bar, Butterfinger, 2.1 oz	4	5	7	8	10
Candy Bar, Chocolate and Almonds, 1.5 oz	3	4	5	6	7
Candy Bar, Chocolate and Rice, 1.5 oz	3	4	5	6	7
Candy Bar, Chunky, 1.4 oz	2	4	5	6	7

THE MEGASTEP VALUE OF FOODS
CANDY *(continued)*

SERVING SIZE: I PIECE, I OUNCE OR I BAR	STEPS/CALORIE				
	<15	16–20	21–25	26–30	>30
Candy Bar, Golden Collection Almond, 2.8 oz	6	8	10	13	15
Candy Bar, Krackel, 1.5 oz	7	10	12	15	18
Candy Bar, Milk Chocolate, 1.5 oz	6	9	12	14	17
Candy Bar, Peanut Bar, 1.4 oz	3	5	6	7	9
Candy Bar, Special Dark, 1.5 oz	3	4	5	6	7
Candy Bar, Whatchamacallit, 1.7 oz	3	4	5	6	7
Caramel Candy Roll, 1 oz	3	4	5	6	8
Chewing Gum, 1 piece	1	1	1	2	2
Chocolate Candy, M&M's Plain, 1.7 oz	3	4	5	6	7
Chocolate, Milk, with Raisins, 1.5 oz	7	10	13	15	18
Chocolate, Semisweet, 1 oz	2	2	3	4	4
Fondant, Sweet Chocolate, 1 large patty	2	3	4	4	5
Fruit Candy, Skittles, 2 oz	3	5	6	7	9
Fruit Candy, Starburst, 2 oz	2	3	4	5	5
Gumdrops, 10 pieces or 1 oz	1	2	2	3	3
Halavah, Plain, 3.5 oz	6	8	11	13	15
Jawbreakers, 6 pieces or 1 oz	1	1	1	2	2
Jellybeans, 1 oz	1	2	2	3	3
Lollipop, 1 piece	0	0	1	1	1
Marshmallow, 1 regular	0	0	1	1	1
Mint Candy, 1 oz	2	3	4	5	5
Mint Candy, After Eight, 1 piece	0	1	1	1	1
Peanut Brittle, 1 oz	2	2	3	4	4
Peanut Butter Cups, Reese's, 1.5 oz	0	1	1	1	1
Peanut Candy, Chocolate Coated, 1 oz	3	4	5	6	7
Peanut Candy, M&M's Peanut, 1.6 oz	3	4	6	7	8
Pecan Candy, Turtles, 1 piece	6	9	11	14	16
Peppermint Mints, 1/2 oz or 3 pieces	1	1	1	2	2
Toffee, Cream, 1 piece	5	8	10	12	14

THE MEGASTEP VALUE OF FOODS
CHIPS AND PRETZELS

SERVING SIZE: I OUNCE	STEPS/CALORIE				
	<15	16–20	21–25	26–30	>30
Cheese Crisps, Cheetos, Curls	2	3	3	4	5
Cheese Crisps, Cheetos, Puffed Balls	2	3	3	4	5
Club Sandwiches, Real Cheese	2	3	4	4	5
Corn Chips, Barbecue	2	3	4	4	5
Corn Chips, Blue Corn, No Added Salt	2	3	3	4	5
Corn Chips, Fritos, Original	2	3	4	4	5
Cornnuts Snack, Nacho	2	2	3	3	4
Crackers, Whole Wheat	1	2	3	3	4
Popcorn, Caramel Coated	2	2	3	3	4
Popcorn, Natural Popcorn Flavor	2	2	3	3	4
Pork Skins, Fried, BBQ Flavored	2	3	4	5	6
Potato Chips, Barbecue	2	3	3	4	5
Potato Chips, Cheese	2	3	3	4	5
Potato Chips, Classic	2	3	3	4	5
Potato Crisps, Cheddar and Sour Cream	2	3	3	4	5
Potato Crisps, Ranch	2	3	3	4	5
Potato Crisps, Sour Cream and Onion	2	3	4	4	5
Potato Sticks	2	3	3	4	5
Pretzel, Soft	2	3	4	5	6
Pretzel, Soft Cheese Filled	5	7	9	11	13
Pretzel, Soft Jalapeño	5	6	8	10	12
Pretzels, Classic Tiny Twists	1	2	3	3	4
Pretzels, Hard, Plain	5	7	9	11	13
Snack Mix, Chex	2	2	3	3	4
Sun Chips, Original	2	3	3	4	5
Taro Chips	1	2	3	3	4
Tortilla Chips, 100% White Corn	2	2	3	4	4
Tortilla Chips, 3D's Nacho Cheesier	2	3	3	4	5
Tortilla Chips, Bite Size	2	3	3	4	5

THE MEGASTEP VALUE OF FOODS
CHIPS AND PRETZELS (continued)

SERVING SIZE: 1 OUNCE	STEPS/CALORIE				
	<15	16–20	21–25	26–30	>30
Tortilla Chips, Ranch	2	3	3	4	5
Trail Mix Snack, Regular	2	3	4	5	6

THE MEGASTEP VALUE OF FOODS
ALCOHOL

SERVING SIZE: AS INDICATED	STEPS/CALORIE				
	<15	16–20	21–25	26–30	>30
Beer, 12 oz Can or Bottle	2	3	3	4	5
Beer, Light, 12 oz Can or Bottle	1	2	3	3	4
MIXED DRINKS, 3 FL OZ					
Bloody Mary	2	2	3	3	4
Brandy Alexander	4	5	7	8	10
Daiquiri	1	2	3	3	4
Gin and Tonic	2	3	4	5	6
Harvey Wallbanger	3	5	6	7	8
Irish Coffee	3	4	5	6	7
Long Island Iced Tea	3	4	5	6	8
Mai Tai	3	5	6	7	9
Manhattan	2	2	3	4	4
Margarita	2	3	4	5	6
Martini	2	3	4	4	5
Piña Colada	3	5	6	7	9
Tequila Sunrise	2	3	4	5	6
Whiskey Sour	2	2	3	4	4
WINE, 4 FL OZ					
Burgundy, Red	1	2	2	2	3

THE MEGASTEP VALUE OF FOODS
ALCOHOL (continued)

			STEPS/CALORIE		
SERVING SIZE: AS INDICATED	<15	16–20	21–25	26–30	>30
Cabernet Sauvignon	1	2	2	2	3
Chablis	1	2	2	2	3
Chianti	1	2	2	3	3
Gewürztraminer	1	2	2	2	3
Riesling	1	2	2	2	3
Rosé Table	1	2	2	2	3
Table	1	2	2	2	3

THE MEGASTEP VALUE OF FOODS
FAST FOODS

			STEPS/CALORIE		
SERVING SIZE: 1 ORDER	<15	16–20	21–25	26–30	>30
BREAKFAST FOODS					
Biscuit with Sausage, Egg and Cheese, *Burger King*	8	11	14	17	20
Biscuit, Bacon Egg and Cheese, *McDonald's*	7	10	12	15	18
Biscuit, Sausage, *McDonald's*	6	8	11	13	16
Breakfast Burrito, *Del Taco*	3	5	6	7	8
Breakfast Platter with Sausage, *Whataburger*	10	14	18	22	26
Breakfast Sandwich, Ham & Egg, *Subway*	4	5	7	8	10
Breakfast Sandwich, Western Egg, *Subway*	4	5	7	8	9
Cinnabuon, Classic	9	13	17	20	24
Croissan'wich with Sausage, Egg & Cheese, *Burger King*	7	10	12	15	17
Egg Mcmuffin, *McDonald's*	4	5	7	8	10
Egg'wich with Bacon & Egg, *Burger King*	5	8	10	12	14
French Toast Sticks with Bacon, *Jack in the Box*	6	8	11	13	16
BEVERAGES					
Chocolate Shake, Junior, *Whataburger*	5	7	8	10	12

THE MEGASTEP VALUE OF FOODS
FAST FOODS (continued)

SERVING SIZE: I ORDER	STEPS/CALORIE				
	<15	16–20	21–25	26–30	>30
Chocolate Shake, Large, *Del Taco*	9	12	16	19	22
Chocolate Shake, Medium, *Burger King*	6	8	10	12	15
Chocolate Shake, Small, *Burger King*	4	6	8	9	11
Frosty, Large, *Wendy's*	7	10	12	15	18
Frosty, Small, *Wendy's*	4	6	8	9	11
Fruizle Express, Berry Lishus, *Subway*	1	2	3	3	4
Fruizle Express, Peach Pizazz, *Subway*	1	2	2	3	3
Fruizle Express, Pineapple Delight, *Subway*	2	2	3	4	4
Fruizle Express, Sunrise Refresher, *Subway*	1	2	3	3	4
McFlurry, Oreo, *McDonald's*	7	10	13	16	19
Milkshake, Chocolate, Medium, *McDonald's*	7	10	13	16	19
Milkshake, Vanilla, Medium, *McDonald's*	6	9	12	14	17
Milkshake, Vanilla, Regular, *Dairy Queen/Brazier*	7	9	12	15	17
Milkshake, Vanilla Malt, Regular, *Dairy Queen/Brazier*	8	11	14	17	20
FRENCH FRIES					
French Fries, Large, *Burger King*	6	9	12	14	17
French Fries, King Size, *Burger King*	8	11	14	17	20
French Fries, Small, *McDonald's*	3	4	5	6	7
French Fries, Medium, *McDonald's*	6	8	10	13	15
French Fries, Large, *McDonald's*	7	10	12	15	18
French Fries, Super Size, *McDonald's*	8	11	14	17	20
French Fries, Medium, *Wendy's*	5	7	9	11	13
French Fries, Biggie, *Wendy's*	6	8	10	12	15
French Fries, Great Biggie, *Wendy's*	7	10	12	15	17
HAMBURGERS					
Cheeseburger, Bacon, *Burger King*	5	7	9	11	13
Cheeseburger, Double Patty, *Burger King*	7	10	13	16	19
Cheeseburger, Double Patty, *Dairy Queen/Brazier*	7	10	13	16	19
Cheeseburger, Double Patty, *Sonic*	8	11	15	18	21

THE MEGASTEP VALUE OF FOODS
FAST FOODS (continued)

SERVING SIZE: 1 ORDER	STEPS/CALORIE				
	<15	16–20	21–25	26–30	>30
Cheeseburger, Double Western Bacon, *Carl's Jr.*	11	16	21	25	30
Cheeseburger, Double Whopper, *Burger King*	13	18	23	28	33
Cheeseburger, Jumbo Jack, *Jack in the Box*	9	12	16	19	22
Cheeseburger, Junior, *Wendy's*	4	6	7	9	11
Cheeseburger, Kid's Meal, *Wendy's*	4	6	7	9	11
Cheeseburger, Quarter Pounder, *McDonald's*	7	10	12	15	17
Cheeseburger, Whopper Jr., *Burger King*	6	8	10	13	15
Hamburger, *Burger King*	4	6	7	9	11
Hamburger, *Dairy Queen/Brazier*	4	6	7	9	10
Hamburger, *Jack in the Box*	4	5	6	8	9
Hamburger, *McDonald's*	3	5	6	8	9
Hamburger, *Rally's*	5	8	10	12	14
Hamburger, *Sonic*	5	7	9	11	13
Hamburger, Big Bacon Classic, *Wendy's*	7	10	13	16	19
Hamburger, Big Mac, *McDonald's*	7	10	13	16	19
Hamburger, Big n' Tasty, *McDonald's*	7	10	12	15	17
Hamburger, Big Xtra!, *McDonald's*	9	13	16	20	23
Hamburger, Double Whopper, *Burger King*	12	17	21	26	30
Hamburger, Jumbo Jack, *Jack in the Box*	7	11	14	17	19
Hamburger, Junior, *Wendy's*	3	5	6	8	9
Hamburger, Justaburger, *Whataburger*	4	5	7	8	10
DESSERTS					
Apple Dessert Pizza, *Pizza Hut*	3	5	6	7	8
Apple Grande Pastry, *Taco John's*	4	5	7	8	10
Cheesecake, Cookies & Creme, *Schlotzsky's Deli*	4	6	8	9	11
Cheesecake, New York Creamstyle, *Schlotzsky's Deli*	4	6	7	9	10
Cheesecake, Strawberry Swirl, *Schlotzsky's Deli*	4	5	7	8	10
Cherry Dessert Pizza, *Pizza Hut*	3	5	6	7	8
Churro Pastry, *Taco John's*	2	2	3	3	4

THE MEGASTEP VALUE OF FOODS
FAST FOODS (continued)

SERVING SIZE: 1 ORDER	STEPS/CALORIE				
	<15	16–20	21–25	26–30	>30
Cini-Minis, *Burger King*	6	8	10	12	15
Cinnamon Bun, *Dunkin' Donuts*	6	9	12	14	17
Cinnamon Roll, *McDonald's*	5	7	9	11	13
Cinnamon Roll, *Whataburger*	4	6	7	9	11
Cinnamon Twists, *Taco Bell*	2	3	3	4	5
Cobbler, Peach, *Hardee's*	4	6	7	9	10
Cookie, Chocolate Chip, *Carl's Jr.*	5	7	9	10	12
Cookie, Chocolate Chip, *McDonald's*	2	3	4	5	6
Cookie, Chocolate Chip, *Schlotzsky's Deli*	2	3	4	4	5
Cookie, Chocolate Chip, *Subway*	3	4	5	6	7
Cookie, Chocolate Chip, *Wendy's*	3	5	6	8	9
Cookie, Chocolate Chocolate Chunk, *Dunkin' Donuts*	3	4	5	6	7
Cookie, M&M, *Subway*	3	4	5	6	7
Cookie, Oatmeal Raisin, *Schlotzsky's Deli*	2	3	3	4	5
Cookie, Oatmeal Raisin, *Subway*	2	4	5	6	7
Cookie, Peanut Butter, *Schlotzsky's Deli*	2	3	4	5	6
Cookie, Peanut Butter, *Subway*	3	4	5	6	7
Cookie, Peanut Butter Chocolate, *Schlotzsky's Deli*	2	3	4	5	6
Cookie, Sugar, *Schlotzsky's Deli*	2	3	4	4	5
Cookie, Sugar, *Subway*	3	4	5	6	7
Cookies, McDonaldland, *McDonald's*	2	3	4	5	6
Croissant, Almond, *Dunkin' Donuts*	4	6	8	10	12
Croissant, Chocolate, *Dunkin' Donuts*	5	7	9	11	13
Danish, Apple, *McDonald's*	4	6	8	10	11
Danish, Cheese, *Carl's Jr.*	5	7	9	11	13
Danish, Cheese, *McDonald's*	5	7	9	11	13
Donut, Apple Crumb, *Dunkin' Donuts*	3	4	5	6	8
Donut, Apple Fritter, *Dunkin' Donuts*	4	5	7	8	10
Donut, Apple n' Spice, *Dunkin' Donuts*	3	4	5	6	7

THE MEGASTEP VALUE OF FOODS

FAST FOODS (continued)

SERVING SIZE: 1 ORDER	STEPS/CALORIE				
	<15	16–20	21–25	26–30	>30
Donut, Bavarian Kreme, *Dunkin' Donuts*	3	4	5	6	7
Donut, Bismark Chocolate Iced, *Dunkin' Donuts*	4	6	8	10	11
Donut, Black Raspberry, *Dunkin' Donuts*	3	4	5	6	7
Donut, Blueberry Cake, *Dunkin' Donuts*	4	5	7	8	10
Donut, Blueberry Crumb, *Dunkin' Donuts*	3	4	6	7	8
Donut, Boston Kreme, *Dunkin' Donuts*	3	4	6	7	8
Donut, Bow Tie, *Dunkin' Donuts*	4	5	7	8	10
Donut, Butternut Cake Ring, *Dunkin' Donuts*	4	5	7	8	10
Donut, Chocolate Cake Glazed, *Dunkin' Donuts*	4	5	7	8	10
Donut, Chocolate Coconut Cake, *Dunkin' Donuts*	4	5	7	8	10
Donut, Chocolate Frosted, *Dunkin' Donuts*	3	4	5	6	7
Donut, Chocolate Kreme Filled, *Dunkin' Donuts*	3	5	6	8	9
Donut, Cinnamon Cake, *Dunkin' Donuts*	3	5	6	8	9
Donut, Coconut Cake, *Dunkin' Donuts*	4	5	7	8	10
Donut, Coffee Roll, *Dunkin' Donuts*	3	5	6	8	9
Donut, Double Chocolate Cake, *Dunkin' Donuts*	4	6	7	9	10
Donut, Dunkin', *Dunkin' Donuts*	3	4	6	7	8
Donut, Eclair, *Dunkin' Donuts*	3	5	6	8	9
Donut, Glazed, *Dunkin' Donuts*	2	3	4	5	6
Donut, Glazed Cake, *Dunkin' Donuts*	3	5	6	8	9
Donut, Glazed Chocolate Cruller, *Dunkin' Donuts*	4	5	6	8	9
Donut, Glazed Cruller, *Dunkin' Donuts*	4	5	7	8	10
Donut, Glazed Fritter, *Dunkin' Donuts*	3	5	6	7	9
Donut, Jelly Filled, *Dunkin' Donuts*	3	4	5	6	7
Donut, Jelly Stick, *Dunkin' Donuts*	4	5	7	8	10
Donut, Lemon, *Dunkin' Donuts*	3	4	5	6	7
Donut, Maple Frosted, *Dunkin' Donuts*	3	4	5	6	7
Donut, Marble Frosted, *Dunkin' Donuts*	3	4	5	6	7
Donut, Old-Fashioned Cake, *Dunkin' Donuts*	3	5	6	7	8

THE MEGASTEP VALUE OF FOODS
FAST FOODS (continued)

SERVING SIZE: I ORDER	STEPS/CALORIE				
	<15	16–20	21–25	26–30	>30
Donut, Plain Cruller, *Dunkin' Donuts*	3	4	6	7	8
Donut, Powdered Cake, *Dunkin' Donuts*	3	5	6	8	9
Donut, Strawberry, *Dunkin' Donuts*	3	4	5	6	7
Donut, Sugar Raised, *Dunkin' Donuts*	2	3	4	5	6
Donut, Toasted Coconut Cake, *Dunkin' Donuts*	4	5	7	8	10
Donut, Vanilla Kreme Filled, *Dunkin' Donuts*	3	5	6	8	9
Donut, Whole Wheat Glazed Cake, *Dunkin' Donuts*	4	6	7	9	10
Munchkin, Cake Plain, *Dunkin' Donuts*	3	4	5	6	7
Pie, Baked Apple, *McDonald's*	3	5	6	7	9
Pie, Dutch Apple, *Burger King*	4	5	7	8	10
Pie, Lemon, *Chick-fil-A*	4	5	6	8	9
Pie, Lemon Meringue, *Krystal*	4	6	8	10	11
Pie, Pecan, *KFC*	6	9	11	14	16
Pie, Pecan, *Krystal*	6	8	10	13	15
Pie, Strawberry Creme, *KFC*	4	5	6	8	9
MEXICAN FOODS					
Bean Burrito, *Taco Bell*	5	7	9	10	12
Beef Burrito, *Taco John's*	4	6	8	10	12
Burrito, Crisp-Bean, *Taco Time*	5	8	10	12	14
Burrito Supreme, *Taco Bell*	5	8	10	12	14
Chalupa Baja, *Taco Bell*	5	7	9	11	13
Chili Cheese Burrito, *Taco Bell*	4	6	8	9	11
Chimichanga, *Taco John's*	6	9	11	14	16
Double Burrito Supreme, *Taco Bell*	6	8	11	13	16
Enchirito, *Taco Bell*	4	6	8	10	12
Fiesta Burrito, *Taco Bell*	5	7	9	10	12
Gordita Baja, *Taco Bell*	4	6	8	10	11
Grilled Stuft Burrito, *Taco Bell*	9	12	16	19	23
Mexican Pizza, *Taco Bell*	5	7	9	11	13

THE MEGASTEP VALUE OF FOODS

FAST FOODS (continued)

SERVING SIZE: 1 ORDER OR AS INDICATED	STEPS/CALORIE				
	<15	16–20	21–25	26–30	>30
Mexican Rice, *Taco Bell*	2	3	4	5	6
Meximelt, *Taco Bell*	4	5	7	8	10
Nachos, *Taco Bell*	4	6	7	9	11
Nachos Bellgrande, *Taco Bell*	10	14	17	21	25
Pintos 'n Cheese, *Taco Bell*	2	3	4	5	6
Quesadilla, Cheese, *Taco Bell*	4	6	8	10	12
Soft Taco Supreme, *Taco Bell*	3	4	6	7	8
Taco, *Taco Bell*	2	3	4	5	6
Taco Salad with Salsa, *Taco Bell*	11	15	20	24	28
Tostada, *Taco Bell*	3	5	6	7	8
PASTA					
Cavatini Pasta, *Pizza Hut*	6	9	11	13	16
Cavatini Supreme Pasta, *Pizza Hut*	7	10	13	16	18
Chicken Parmesan Noodles, *Mazzio's Pizza*	7	11	14	17	19
Fettuccine Noodles, Alfredo, *Mazzio's Pizza*	6	8	10	12	15
Meat, Lasagna, Small, *Mazzio's Pizza*	6	8	11	13	15
Spaghetti Entrée, Marinara, *Big Boy*	6	8	10	13	15
Spaghetti Entrée, Meat, *Shakey's Pizza*	12	17	22	26	31
Spaghetti Entrée, Small, *Mazzio's Pizza*	4	5	7	8	10
Spaghetti with Marinara Sauce, *Pizza Hut*	6	9	11	14	16
Spaghetti with Meatballs, *Pizza Hut*	11	15	20	24	28
Spaghetti with Meat Sauce, *Pizza Hut*	8	11	14	17	20
PIZZA 1 slice					
Cheese Pizza, Big New Yorker, *Pizza Hut*	5	7	9	11	13
Cheese Pizza, Deep Dish, *Domino's Pizza*	7	11	14	17	20
Cheese Pizza, Golden Crust, *Godfather's Pizza*	3	5	6	7	9
Cheese Pizza, Hand Tossed, *Domino's Pizza*	6	9	12	14	17
Cheese Pizza, Hand Tossed, *Pizza Hut*	4	6	7	9	10
Cheese Pizza, Personal Pan, *Pizza Hut*, 1 pie	10	15	19	23	27

THE MEGASTEP VALUE OF FOODS
FAST FOODS (continued)

SERVING SIZE: AS INDICATED	STEPS/CALORIE				
	<15	16–20	21–25	26–30	>30
Cheese Pizza, Sicilian, *Pizza Hut*	4	5	7	8	10
Cheese Pizza, Stuffed Crust, *Pizza Hut*	6	8	10	12	15
Chicken Supreme Pizza, Hand Tossed, *Pizza Hut*	4	5	7	8	10
Ham Pizza, Hand Tossed, *Pizza Hut*	3	5	6	8	9
Italian Sausage Pizza, Hand Tossed, *Pizza Hut*	5	7	8	10	12
Meat Lover's Pizza, Hand Tossed, *Pizza Hut*	5	7	9	11	12
Pepperoni Lover's Pizza, Hand Tossed, *Pizza Hut*	5	7	9	10	12
Pepperoni Pizza, Big New Yorker, *Pizza Hut*	5	7	9	11	13
Pizza, Hawaiian, *Papa Murphy's*	4	5	7	8	10
Pizza, Murphy's Combo, *Papa Murphy's*	4	6	8	10	12
Pizza, Vegetarian, *Papa Murphy's*	4	6	7	9	10
Super Supreme Pizza, Hand Tossed, *Pizza Hut*	4	6	8	10	12
Taco Pizza, Beef, Hand Tossed, *Pizza Hut*	3	5	6	8	9
Veggie Lover's Pizza, Hand Tossed, *Pizza Hut*	4	5	6	8	9
SANDWICHES, 1 sandwich					
Albacore Tuna Sandwich, *Schlotzsky's Deli*	13	18	23	28	33
Barbecue Chicken Sandwich, *Carl's Jr.*	4	5	6	8	9
Barbecue Sandwich, Arby-Q, *Arby's*	5	7	9	11	13
Batter-dipped Fish Sandwich, *Long John Silver's*	4	6	7	9	11
Beef Barbecue Sandwich, *Dairy Queen/Brazier*	3	4	5	6	7
BLT Sandwich, *Sonic*	4	6	8	9	11
Cheese Sandwich, Grilled, *Sonic*	4	5	7	8	10
Chick 'n Crisp Sandwich, *Burger King*	6	8	11	13	15
Chicken Bacon 'n Swiss Sandwich, *Arby's*	8	11	14	17	20
Chicken Caesar Pita, *Wendy's*	6	9	11	14	16
Chicken Club Sandwich, *Carl's Jr.*	6	8	11	13	15
Chicken McGrill Sandwich, *McDonald's*	6	8	10	13	15
Chicken Sandwich, *Burger King*	9	13	16	20	23
Chicken Sandwich, *Chick-fil-A*	4	5	7	8	10

THE MEGASTEP VALUE OF FOODS

FAST FOODS (continued)

SERVING SIZE: I SANDWICH	STEPS/CALORIE				
	<15	16–20	21–25	26–30	>30
Chicken Sandwich, Original Recipe, *KFC*	6	8	10	13	15
Corn Dog, *Sonic*, one	4	5	6	8	9
Crispy Chicken Sandwich, *McDonald's*	7	10	13	15	18
Croissan'wich with Sausage and Cheese, *Burger King*	6	8	10	13	15
Filet-o-Fish Sandwich, *McDonald's*	6	8	11	13	16
Fish Sandwich, *Arthur Treacher's*	6	8	10	12	15
Fish Sandwich, BK Big, *Burger King*	9	13	17	20	24
Fish Sandwich, Ultimate, *Long John Silver's*	5	8	10	12	14
French Dip Sub, *Arby's*	6	9	11	14	16
Garden Ranch Chicken Pita, *Wendy's*	6	9	11	13	16
Garden Veggie Pita, *Wendy's*	5	7	9	11	13
Ham and Cheese Sandwich, *Pizza Hut*	7	10	13	15	18
Ham Sandwich, Deli Style, *Subway*	2	3	4	5	6
Hot Dog, *Dairy Queen/Brazier*	6	9	11	13	16
Hot Dog with Cheese, *Dairy Queen/Brazier*	7	10	12	15	18
Hot Dog with Chili, *Dairy Queen/Brazier*	7	10	13	16	19
Market Fresh Roast Beef and Swiss, *Arby's*	10	15	19	23	27
Market Fresh Roast Chicken Caesar, *Arby's*	10	15	19	23	27
Market Fresh Roast Ham and Swiss, *Arby's*	9	13	17	20	24
Market Fresh Turkey and Swiss, *Arby's*	10	14	17	21	25
Market Fresh Turkey Ranch and Bacon, *Arby's*	11	16	20	25	29
Market Fresh Ultimate BLT, *Arby's*	10	15	19	23	27
Pastrami and Swiss Sandwich, *Schlotzsky's Deli*	21	30	39	47	55
Philly Sandwich, *Schlotzsky's Deli*	21	31	39	48	56
Roast Beef and Cheese Sandwich, *Schlotzsky's Deli*	22	31	40	49	58
Roast Beef Sandwich, Big, *Hardee's*	5	7	9	11	14
Roast Beef Sandwich, Deli Style, *Subway*	3	4	5	6	7
Roast Chicken Club, *Arby's*	7	10	12	15	18
Spicy Chicken Sandwich, *Wendy's*	5	7	9	11	14

THE MEGASTEP VALUE OF FOODS
FAST FOODS (continued)

SERVING SIZE: I SANDWICH	STEPS/CALORIE				
	<15	16–20	21–25	26–30	>30
Sub, 6" Cold Cut Trio, *Subway*	5	7	10	12	14
Sub, 6" Ham, *Subway*	3	5	6	7	9
Sub, 6" Italian BMT, *Subway*	6	8	10	13	15
Sub, 6" Meatball, *Subway*	6	9	12	14	17
Sub, 6" Roast Beef, *Subway*	3	5	6	7	9
Sub, 6" Roasted Chicken Breast, *Subway*	4	6	7	9	10
Sub, 6" Seafood & Crab, *Subway*	5	7	9	11	12
Sub, 6" Tuna, *Subway*	5	8	10	12	14
Sub, 6" Turkey Breast, *Subway*	3	5	6	7	8
Sub, 6" Turkey Breast and Ham, *Subway*	3	5	6	7	9
Sub, 6" Veggie Delite, *Subway*	3	4	5	6	7
Tuna Sandwich, Deli Style, *Subway*	4	6	7	9	10

Useful Resources for Weight Management

America on the Move. This is a grassroots national weight-gain prevention initiative offered by a nonprofit group, the Partnership to Promote Healthy Eating and Active Living. The Web site www.americaonthe move.org offers tips for simple ways to cut 100 calories from your diet and simple ways to increase your steps. You can buy a step counter here and keep track of your daily LifeSteps. You can sign up for free to join America on the Move and find out about activities in your local area.

The Robert Wood Johnson Foundation promotes active living. Visit their Web site at www.rwjf.org to learn more.

Centers for Obesity Research and Education. This is a group formed to teach health care professionals about weight management. Visit them at www.uchsc.edu/core.

International Food Information Council has a great Web site to educate children and their parents about nutrition and physical activity. Visit www.kidnetic.com.

Cooper Clinic. The Cooper Clinic promotes healthy and active living. Visit them at www.cooperinstitute.org.

Colorado Weigh. This is a commercial weight-management program developed at the University of Colorado Health Sciences Center. The program uses many of the strategies discussed in *The Step Diet Book.* Visit them at www.coloradoweigh.com.

The following government agencies offer Web sites that contain useful information about weight management:

National Institute of Diabetes & Digestive and Kidney Diseases. www.niddk.nih.gov

National Heart, Lung, and Blood Institute. www.nhlbi.nih.gov

Centers for Disease Control and Prevention. www.cdc.gov

U.S. Department of Agriculture. www.usda.gov

World Health Organization. www.who.int

The following professional organizations offer useful information about weight management:

American Dietetic Association. www.eatright.org

American Diabetes Association. www.diabetes.org

American Heart Association. www.americanheart.org

North American Association for the Study of Obesity. www.naaso.org

American College of Sports Medicine. www.acsm.org

These are some books that may be helpful in understanding more about why we gain weight:

Fat Land by Greg Critser

Volumetrics by Barbara Rolls, Ph.D., and Robert A. Barnett

Fight Fat After Forty by Pamela Peeke, M.D.

Index

A

Alcohol, 134, 139–40
  MegaStep value for, 260–61
Appearance, concern for, 56
Appetite, 29, 80, 125
Aqua jogging, 118
Artificial sweeteners, 139
Asian foods, MegaStep value for, 244
Atkins diet, 136

B

Balance:
  in all aspects of life, 129, 158
  see also Energy balance
Basketball, 96
Beef, 169
  MegaStep value for, 238–39
Behavior:
  creating a new identity and, 158
  establishing healthier habits and, 78
  impact of environment on, 59–62
  interaction of genes and, 59
  making small changes in, xvii,
    25–26, 30, 32
Beverages:
  fast-food, MegaStep value for,
    261–62
  free foods, 85
  75 percent strategy and, 82, 83, 86
  tips for, 170–72
Biking, 37, 98–99
Birch, Leann, 23, 101
Blood pressure, 50, 53, 54
Body mass index (BMI), 45–51
  calcium and, 178

categories of, 46–47
  health risks and, 47–51
  tables for, 48–49
  waist circumference and, 52–53
BodySteps, 68–69
  calculating, 69–71, 112–13
BodySteps tables, 140, 179–235
  for men, 208–35
  for women, 180–207
Body temperature, thermic effect of
    food and, 143
Breakfast:
  maintaining weight loss and, 120,
    129
  MegaStep value for foods eaten at,
    237, 261
  75 percent strategy and, 86, 120
  tips for, 166
Brownies, MegaStep value for, 248

C

Cajun foods, MegaStep value for, 245
Cakes, MegaStep value for, 248–49
Calcium, 178
Calorie-modified foods, 138–39
Calories (energy):
  body's ability to burn, 140–44
  burning 100 additional, per day,
    31–42
  counting, 8, 91, 108
  energy density of foods and, 134–40
  steps per (tables), 68, 72–75
  stored in body, 18, 132–33, 145
  weight gain from 100 extra, per day,
    17–18
Cancer, x–xi, 47, 50, 51, 53

HOW TO USE YOUR STEP DIET PEDOMETER

It is very important that you wear your step counter correctly if you are to get an accurate reading. You'll find directions for use on page 2, but here are some important things to keep in mind:

• All people are built differently, so the best place to mount your counter may be different for you than for other people. For starters, try clipping it on your waistband. If your waistband is flimsy, try clipping it to your underwear. Many women wear their pedometers clipped to the middle of their bras. Make sure to attach the strap (found in the box, under the pedometer) and use it, both to prevent breakage (from sudden impact if dropped) and loss.

• Make sure you've pressed the reset button so that you're starting at 0, and then walk 100 steps. If your pedometer reads between 90 and 110, it is working, and you are wearing it properly. If your reading is less than 90 or more than 110 (or if you just want to try to get the reading as close to 100 as possible), move the pedometer to another spot on your waistband, reset it, and walk 100 steps. Keep moving the pedometer around until you get a reading between 90 and 110. If you have a bigger belly, it's possible that you'll get a more accurate reading by mounting the pedometer on your back waistband. In general, the best placement is as close to the body, on either your waist or torso, as you can get it. You want the pedometer to "feel" your footsteps through your body.

• Wear the step counter as horizontally straight as possible, and no more than five degrees off the vertical. If it is tilted, it will probably undercount. Older people who may walk softly or shuffle their feet can also experience undercounting. If that is the situation for you, just remember that the most critical thing is that you increase your steps, even if that increase is relative. Overcounting is more rare, and usually occurs when you are doing something that involves bouncing, such as riding in a golf cart.

• Remember that your step counter is *always on*. You need to hold the reset button with the flat end of your finger—and not a pointed fingernail—if you want to start a new count.

WHAT TO DO IF YOU THINK YOUR STEP COUNTER ISN'T WORKING

• Go through all of the steps listed above to make sure you are wearing your pedometer correctly. These devices have a very low defect rate, and 99 percent of difficulties are caused by wearing them where the internal pendulum mechanism cannot function properly.

• Send your service questions to the manufacturer, Accusplit, Inc., by e-mail at service@accusplit.com, or by mail to the address below.

• If you are sure you are not experiencing a "wearing position" problem, if your step counter does not display at all, or if the display is distorted, please return the pedometer for a no-cost replacement. But it is crucial that you check your wearing position first; if that is the problem, getting a new pedometer will not make it go away.

• The step counters are not warrantied to be waterproof, though they are protected against rain and sweat. If your unit gets soaked, try drying it with a blow dryer. It may continue to work. If not, you should purchase a replacement (see below).

• Replacement batteries are also not covered by the warranty. The battery that comes with your step counter should last between two and three years. If it needs to be replaced, buy an L1142 button battery or equivalent, at most grocery, drug, or hardware stores. The small back cover under the clip covers the battery, and can be easily pried off.

• If your step counter needs to be refurbished, replaced, or repaired within one year of purchase because of defects in manufacture (the extent of the warranty), return it, along with a copy of your dated store receipt (as proof of purchase), your daytime phone number, and your address to

AST Repair Center
2290A Ringwood Avenue
San Jose, California 95131

• If your step counter needs to be refurbished, replaced, or repaired more than one year after purchase, return it to the AST Repair Center, along with your daytime phone number, address, and a $5.00 shipping and handling fee.

• If you want to order additional step counters for yourself or your family, go to the Web site for America on the Move: www.americaonthemove.org. This nonprofit organization, dedicated to getting people to add more steps to their days, will be happy to fill your order.

Happy walking!